Belly Button
HEALING

UNLOCKING YOUR SECOND BRAIN FOR A HEALTHY LIFE

Belly Button
HEALING

ILCHI LEE

BEST
LIFE
MEDIA

459 N. Gilbert Rd. Suite C-210
Gilbert, AZ 85234
www.BestLifeMedia.com
(480) 926-2480

Please understand that this book is not intended to treat, cure, or prevent any disease or illness. The information in this book is intended for educational purposes only, not as medical advice. Always check with your health professional before changing your diet, eating, or health program. The author and publisher disclaim any liability arising directly or indirectly from the use and application of any of the book's contents.

Second paperback edition: February 2019
Library of Congress Control Number: 2016941961
ISBN: 978-1-935127-91-8

Photo Permissions Acknowledgments
Page 14 © iStock.com/blackjake; Cover, Page 148 © iStock.com/PeopleImages

If you don't take care of your body,
where are you going to live?

—UNKNOWN

Table of Contents

INTRODUCTION

Take an Interest in Your Belly Button

For the past 36 years, I have been exploring different ways of helping people achieve an optimal state of well-being. All of these methods are designed to maximize the natural healing powers of the human body, and they combine the principles and methods of Eastern energy study with modern brain science. My programs include familiar, basic methods, such as breathing, meditation, qigong, yoga, and energy healing, as well as more unique exercises, such as Brain Wave Vibration and LifeParticle training. Collectively, these methods comprise my Brain Education five-step program, which is designed to maximize the human brain's potential.

During the process of creating these methods, my mind was focused on just one question: How can I create an easy and simple method that anyone can quickly learn and benefit from? From the answers I've found, I've developed many mind-body training methods that are extremely effective, but that can be learned by anyone with a minute to spare. For example, Brain Wave Vibration stabilizes brain waves and improves focus with just simple shaking of the head, and Toe Tapping improves energy and blood circulation, and relaxes the whole body as one taps the toes together.

In the process of researching principles and methods for healing the human body, I have developed a keen interest in the belly button. I first noticed the potential of the belly button when I developed digestive troubles. When I massaged my abdomen and pressed my belly button, I discovered that my stomachaches stopped. Additionally, when I pushed specific areas of my belly button after I hurt my lower back, I found that it relieved my pain, allowing me to recover more rapidly.

Based on these experiences, I began teaching Belly Button Healing whenever I met people who needed help with their health. Particularly in my retreats and workshops over the last several years, I've used pain points found around the navel to determine the physical state of participants who were having health problems. After applying Belly Button Healing methods, many participants found relief or even complete reversal of their symptoms. That is why I felt the need to write this book—so that everyone can get a similar benefit.

Many people, unable to manage their own health, rely on drugs, hospitals, or specialists. We certainly should get help from specialists when we need it, but our first line of defense should be our bodies' natural healing ability. This means adopting a healthy lifestyle that strengthens our vitality and immunity. The tips you'll discover in this book are meant to accentuate the benefits of other healthy habits, such as sufficient exercise and a balanced diet.

A Way to Become Closer to Yourself

Belly Button Healing is also a way to become closer to yourself. If you do Belly Button Healing for a while, you'll deepen your understanding of your own body. You'll become more aware of where you feel pain in your body, where you feel cold or warm, and whether your energy and blood are circulating well. You will begin to notice the depth and length of your breathing, and whether your mind and body are relaxed. As you experiment with experiences like these, you will feel the changes that come with doing Belly Button Healing. You will be able to communicate with your body, and you will learn how you should manage and care for it. Additionally, through deep Belly Button Breathing, you will experience your own life energy, along with deep stability and peace, as you are connected with the Source of life.

In our times, personal relationships are growing more difficult. Belly Button Healing, however, is a simple way to become closer to other people. You can teach it to the people around you, and your family members can take turns performing Belly Button Healing on each other. It is as simple and as fun as playing a game together. Trust and bonds of affection naturally grow deeper between the person giving and the person receiving Belly Button Healing through the healing power of touch. And you might communicate more readily with each other as you talk about how you are changing from Belly Button Healing.

Beyond Self-Healing

I hope that as you share Belly Button Healing, it will spread widely as an approach to health that we can practice in our daily lives, as a method of true healing that links mind to mind and heart to heart, instead of remaining at the level of self-healing. What we feel as we heal each other—pure love that wishes for the other person to become healthier and happier—is our starting point for healing ourselves and our relationships. Looking at the bigger picture, I believe that this is the secret for healing our suffering world. When people with such hearts come together, they will be able to heal society and the Earth.

People who want to care for others in the way they care for themselves are gathering to take part in a global Earth Citizen Movement. I earnestly hope that Belly Button Healing will be used actively as a simple, yet powerful method to promote health, and to heal the Earth. Belly Button Healing is a truly powerful tool that not only lets anyone experience immediate effects, but allows them, through deep breathing, to experience their deep inner nature. There is hardly anyone in this world without a navel. Few people, however, know the true significance of the belly button. The navel, which contains the amazing principles of life, is a button for promoting natural healing and vitality, a button through which we can connect with people and the world.

Take an interest in your belly button, starting right now, at this moment. Press your belly button whenever you get the chance. Experience a deeper connection with yourself through your belly button. Profound, holistic healing and transformation will begin in the center of your body, which will in turn spread to your whole life and to the whole world.

April 2016
Ilchi Lee

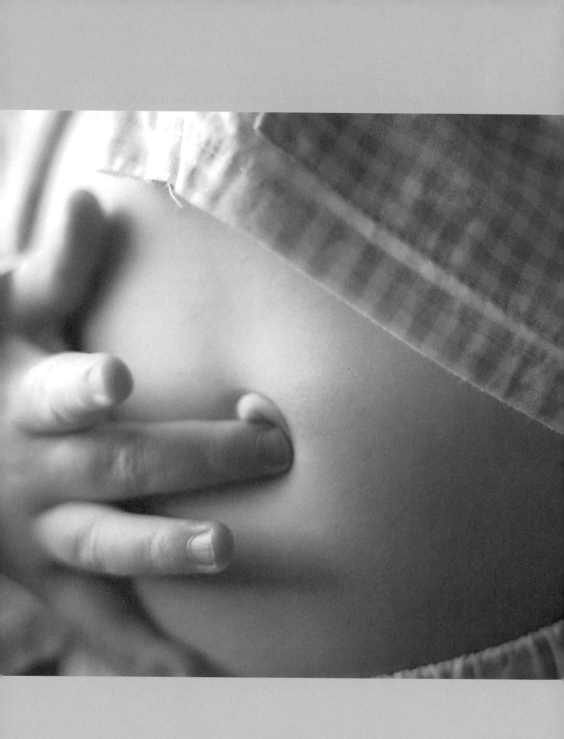

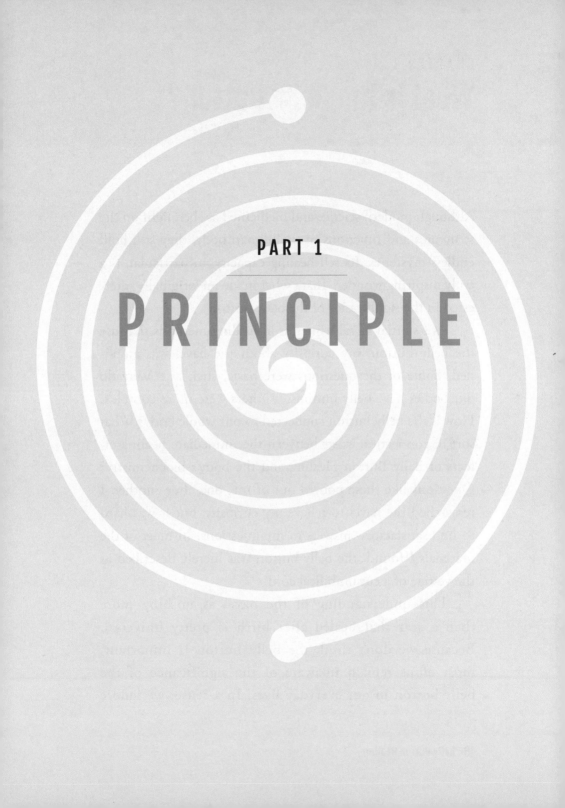

PART 1

PRINCIPLE

CHAPTER 1

What Is the Belly Button?

Although modern science and medicine has shed light on the structures and functions of the human body, they still hold endless mysteries. Its self-healing capacity, in particular, is a truly inspiring wonder. That's what made me originally interested in the significance of the belly button.

As I started to take interest in healing methods that use the belly button, my curiosity about the navel was amplified. Some of the questions were basic, such as, "Why do our bodies have belly buttons?" Others were more complex: How is the belly button connected to our whole body? What sort of connection exists between the immediate healing effects of Belly Button Healing and the body's biochemistry? Questions like these poured out of me, one after another. I researched the navel to relieve my curiosity, but it was hard to find satisfactory answers to my questions. In most of the materials I found, the belly button was merely described as the vestige of a cut umbilical cord.

This understanding of the navel as nothing more than a scar that healed after birth is pretty universal. Because we don't think the belly button is important, most of us remain unaware of the significance of the belly button in our everyday lives. In a sense, we ignore the belly button as if it weren't even there.

We hold slight differences in our attitudes toward the belly button, depending on our region, culture, and era. In Western cultures, people have always been taught that they should thoroughly wash a baby's belly button, but, in Korea where I grew up, adults taught children not to touch the navel. On seeing children having fun picking foreign matter out of their belly buttons, Korean adults would stop them, saying, "You'll get a bellyache if you pick your navel."

Until only a few decades ago, it was considered taboo to show your belly button in most Eastern and Western cultures. The few exceptions include places like India, where traditional dress reveals the navel, and the Middle East, where the belly dance is traditional. In modern times, though, exposing the navel is fashionable and is considered natural. Young people, overflowing with healthy beauty, wear sportswear that reveals the navel. This attire is generally viewed positively and, on occasion, even with envy. These days, the belly button is becoming an object of fashion and ornamentation, so much so that there is even cosmetic surgery for the navel and belly-button piercing.

Unknown Secrets of the Belly Button

Is the belly button really nothing more than a birth scar that no longer has any use except for decoration? Whenever I look at my navel, I can't help thinking, "There must be some unknown use for the belly button, something associated with the body's system . . ." As I've continued to meet countless people in the process of applying the Belly Button Healing method I've devised, I came to believe that the belly button holds yet-unknown secrets for recovering and maintaining health.

The principles and methods of the Belly Button Healing introduced in this book grew out of my intuitive insights about the importance of the belly button. My 35 years of study of the natural healing power of the human body and mind, combined with recent scientific research on the human body, especially research on the gut, played important roles in further developing the method.

I've learned that, more than the thousands of microbes living inside our belly button itself, the real wonders of the navel lie in what's behind it. In that important area of your body, its center, we find yards of intestines, major blood vessels, important lymph nodes, trillions of gut microbes, a strong line of immune defense, and most of all, our second brain—the enteric nervous system.

The health of this microecosystem affects the health of our whole body. That health is highly dependent on circulation and temperature. We thrive when we keep the world behind our navel warm and flowing, something that's difficult to do in today's modern, sedentary lifestyle. Without much effort, Belly Button Healing stokes a fire in our belly, realigns our body structure for better flow, flushes waste, and pumps vitality to the entire body.

In the first part of this book, I detail how Belly Button Healing accomplishes this from three different angles. The first is from a physical perspective based on the systems of the human body as they are currently understood by modern science. The second is from an energetic perspective, which is based on Eastern medical principles and systems of energy. The third is from a philosophical perspective based on my realizations concerning the source of life and our connection with the earth through the belly button.

In the second part, I describe the practice of Belly Button Healing step-by-step, showing you how to perform it on yourself and other people. I also go into detail about a few abdominal exercises you can do to complement your healing practice. I hope that with this accessible self-healing method, vibrant, holistic health and a broader awakening to who you are become normal parts of your life.

CHAPTER 2
The Physical Perspective

When a child is born, the cutting of the umbilical cord is usually treated with some cultural significance. Even in today's high-tech delivery rooms, the father is often given that privilege, and it symbolizes the child's entrance into the world as a separate individual. But beyond that first day of life, we don't think of it as having much significance. This is not really correct, however, since most of its physical structures remain within our bodies after its prenatal function has ended. Understanding this can help you get to know yourself and how you came to be in this world.

As it is generally known, the belly button is a vestige of the umbilical cord. The umbilical cord was the lifeline that allowed us to develop as a living being. In the womb, the fetus receives a supply of oxygen, nutrients, and information through its umbilical connection with its mother's placenta. One umbilical vein and two umbilical arteries flow through the umbilical cord. Through these, we receive plenty of blood from our mother's placenta, and we send carbon dioxide and waste products out.

The vessels that bring blood to and from the fetus, as well as other ducts that remove waste, constrict and degenerate into ligaments after birth. These ligaments extend from the

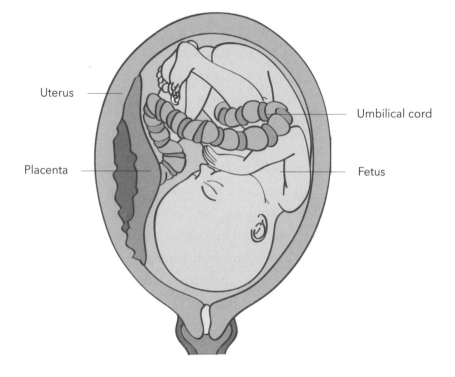

Uterus

Placenta

Umbilical cord

Fetus

THE HISTORY OF YOUR BELLY BUTTON

navel to the liver and bladder. Some remain embedded in the abdominal wall behind the navel. The inner portions of the umbilical artery remain a part of the circulatory system, connecting to the internal iliac artery that goes down into the legs, as well as the arteries that supply blood to the upper part of the bladder and ureter. Additionally, what was the allantoic duct during the fetal period atrophies and connects the belly button to the upper part of the bladder.

Have you ever had a tingling sensation in your bladder or urinary system or felt an urge to urinate when you washed, picked, or poked your belly button? This is because by stimulating your belly button, you also stimulate your umbilical vein and allantoic duct which are connected from your navel to your bladder. The functions of the vessels have changed because your umbilical cord was cut, but their structure remains. That's why pressing and massaging your belly button, which once acted as a port and hub supplying oxygen and nutrients received from your umbilical cord to your whole body, has great significance. When you do Belly Button Healing, the stimulation can affect the liver, bladder, pelvis, and legs, because they are connected with those former umbilical vessels.

The key to Belly Button Healing, I've discovered, is found in the position of the belly button. The navel is in the center of the human body. Gathered around the belly button are major organs for maintaining life, including digestive, circulatory, respiratory, and immune organs. Consequently,

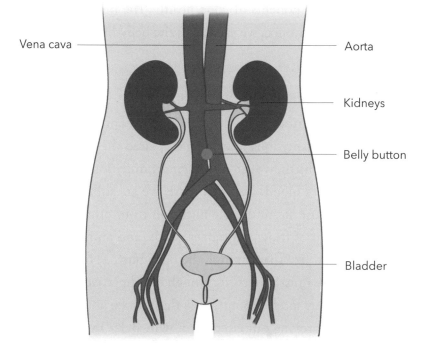

Vena cava

Aorta

Kidneys

Belly button

Bladder

CIRCULATORY AND URINARY ORGANS
AROUND YOUR BELLY BUTTON

we can influence these organs through Belly Button Healing. Promoting good digestion, facilitating blood circulation, breathing deeply, and strengthening the immune system are essential components of good health The button that turns these on all at once, we can say, is the belly button.

Speed Up Your Blood Circulation

The belly button area of the abdomen continues to be the source of vitality long after we have exited the womb. As you know, after birth, we can no longer get nutrition directly from our mother's blood. But, in a sense, we are still not independent, because we must take nutrition from other organisms, in the form of fruits, vegetables, seeds, and animal products. We do not take that through the belly button, of course, but instead, we must process it through our digestive tract, which converts our food into nutrients that can be absorbed by the blood. Improving our circulation with Belly Button Healing can help us get the most out of the food that we eat.

The organ that is stimulated directly when you press your belly button is your small intestine. The intestines are the organs that handle key digestive functions. When food mixed with gastric fluid goes from the stomach into the small intestine, it is broken down into smaller particles and its nutrients digested, and the remains are sent to the large intestine. Occupying virtually all of the central abdomen, the small intestine reaches a length of approximately 23 feet (seven meters).

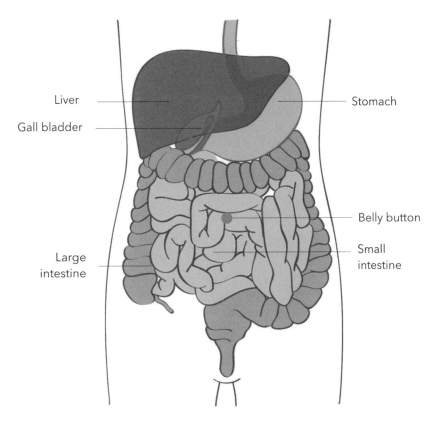

Liver

Gall bladder

Stomach

Belly button

Small intestine

Large intestine

DIGESTIVE ORGANS AROUND YOUR BELLY BUTTON

The large intestine is usually about five feet (1.5 meters), so, combined, the approximately 28-foot-long small and large intestines fill the abdomen.

Protruding from the walls of the small intestine are tightly packed intestinal villi, which absorb nutrients. The inner wall of the small intestine is wrinkled as much as possible to increase its surface area, so much so that a thousand microscopic villi are attached to a single cell. If we combine the surface area of all these villi, they are approximately 3200 square feet (300 square meters) in size.

Nutrients absorbed by the villi move into the capillaries of the small intestine and are transported throughout the body. The cells use these nutrients to create plenty of energy, which makes the body warm and vital.

To perform this important job, about 30 to 40 percent of your body's entire blood volume flows through the abdominal organs. The thickest blood vessels in our bodies, the abdominal aorta and inferior vena cava, are located immediately behind the belly button. You can feel your pulse beating strongly if you gently press your navel with your hand. This is your pulse felt through your abdominal aorta. Because of its position, by pressing and stimulating your belly button, you can increase the blood circulation in the abdominal area most effectively.

Usually, it takes 45 seconds for blood to circulate through our bodies one time. As you press down repeatedly and rhythmically during Belly Button Healing, the small intestine moves more vigorously, improving the flow of blood in the small intestine and throughout the body. It also warms the area, which is known to assist blood circulation.

Make Your Gut Brain Happy

You may have heard people use phrases that connect the mind and the emotions to the gut, such as "you have to have guts to do that" or "I have butterflies in my stomach." Well, as it turns out, science has discovered that the neurons that manage your gut from esophagus to anus, the enteric nervous system (ENS), can operate independently from your brain. Just like your brain, it has cells that take in information, cells that process it, and cells that tell your digestive system what to do. Even if the connection between the enteric nervous system and the brain is cut, or your brain stops working, the gut keeps functioning. When the gut ceases to function, though, the brain also ceases to function. That's why the ENS and its related cells are called "the second brain," or "the gut brain."

The brain and the gut brain come from the same embryonic tissue during development. The gut brain matures much earlier than the brain, however. The vitally important ENS is fully functional at birth, while the brain continues to mature even into the teenage years.

In fact, the ENS has the most cells of any part of the nervous system outside the brain. While the brains in our heads have about 100 billion cells, the gut brain has about 300 to

500 million—about five times the number in the spinal cord. The function of our gut is so important that it has a direct line to the brain via a cranial nerve called the vagus nerve. There are over 2,000 neural fibers connecting our brains with our gut brains. Through this close connection, these two brains can communicate closely and rapidly. The ENS can tell the brain what's going on in our guts and the brain, the body's master control, can send signals so that the digestive system can work together with the rest of the body. That's why, when a problem develops in the intestines, it affects the brain immediately, and, conversely, when a problem develops in the brain, problems develop in the intestines. Have you ever had a stomachache or indigestion when you heard bad news or were nervous? Have you ever had a headache when you had gas or constipation? These cases show us the tight connection between the intestines and the brain.

The influence of our gut brain on the conditions and functioning of our head brain goes even deeper. For example, the neurons and hormone-producing cells in the gut generate chemical signals that affect our emotions. Approximately 50 percent of our dopamine, the neurotransmitter that enables us to feel happiness, is created in the gut brain. Over 90 percent of our serotonin, the neurotransmitter that gives us feelings of well-being, is also created in the gut, while only three percent is made in our brains.

Serotonin affects your mood, appetite, sleep, sexual desire and function, memory and learning, and social behavior.

Depression and anxiety, which develop when we don't have enough serotonin, may be strongly influenced by problems of the intestines. Consequently, improving the health of the intestines can increase serotonin secretion, enabling us to maintain a positive mood and causing us to feel satisfaction and motivation.

In traditional Eastern medicine, it is said that "clear intestines make a clear brain," emphasizing the importance of gut health for overall well-being. And the intestines are believed to handle "emotional" digestion. Emotions like anxiety, anger, and fear cause contraction of the intestines, reducing intestinal function. By releasing tension in the intestines, according to energy theory, it is possible to release undigested, stagnated emotions.

In addition to our emotions, our gut health has other effects on our brains. Most children with conditions like ADHD or autism have issues with their gut. Some adult brain conditions, such as Alzheimer's disease, have been found to have a strong correlation with gut condition, too. Researchers have found that adults over age fifty with symptoms of depression caused by serotonin deficiency were twice as likely to develop vascular dementia and 65 percent more likely to develop Alzheimer's disease than similarly aged people who weren't depressed. Many of these brain conditions have been shown to get better when the patient's gut condition improved. Sometimes, this was more effective than traditional treatments that target the brain directly.

The intestines coil in a counterclockwise direction, centered on the belly button, where the most nerves are also distributed. Your nerves are activated when you press your belly button with gentle and rhythmic movements. Then, when you stop this motion, your nerves instantly relax, bringing further release of tension in the intestines and relaxation of body and mind. The belly button works like a trigger point to stimulate the entire ENS. Additionally, while you're doing Belly Button Healing, you focus on exhaling. Focused exhalation increases the activity of the parasympathetic nervous system, which helps your body to establish a more relaxed, resting state ideal for the health of your gut.

Maximize Your Immune Power

When you are in your mother's womb, your immune system comes entirely from your mother, as she shares her antibodies with you through her blood. But as we enter the world on our own, we must develop and maintain our own immune systems. This system is of great concern for people's health these days, since immune diseases are on the rise and the incidence of other diseases, such as cancer and various viral diseases, could be reduced if people's immunity were stronger. Here again, most people do not realize how important their belly button is to their health.

Large lymph nodes, called abdominal lymph nodes, are concentrated around the belly button. Lymph nodes are organs of the immune system. Just as blood vessels are distributed throughout the body, so, too, lymphatic vessels are spread throughout the body. Lymphatic fluid, which contains immune cells, flows along these vessels, collecting waste material. Lymph nodes, the points where lymphatic vessels connect, handle immune reactions, such as inspecting lymphatic fluid and creating antibodies. Many of these lymph nodes are gathered around the navel, as if surrounding it. Belly Button Healing assists immune reaction and excretion of waste products by appropriately stimulating these lymph nodes to facilitate the flow of lymphatic fluid.

When you talk about the immune system, people generally think of leukocytes and lymphocytes fighting against antigens that have entered the body. Intestinal health, in fact, has an important impact on immunity to disease because many immune cells are distributed in the gut, which has a lot of blood. Immunity, however, does not signify only the activity of immune cells. Recently, observers see the immune function of enteric microbes as equally important as that of immune cells.

Our bodies have what scientists call a "torus structure," where a single channel extends from the mouth to the anus. In this hollow tube, different substances, including food, entering from the outside come into direct contact with the membranes of the gastrointestinal tract, or, in other words, with the body's inner skin. The body's internal skin, just like its external skin, is directly exposed to outside substances.

When they enter the body, external substances stay for a short time in the mouth and esophagus, but they remain for a long period inside the intestines. During this time, the microbes in our gut protect our bodies from harmful yeast and bacteria.

The microbes living in the intestines also affect intestinal immunity. Three hundred to 1,000 species of microbes live in the intestines, and this environment is referred to as "gut microbiota." Their total weight is approximately two to four pounds, and about 60 percent of fecal weight is made up of such microbes. Gut microbes not only break down food and create vitamins and hormones, but they also act to stop pathogens. Intestinal microbes are generally classified as beneficial bacteria, intermediate bacteria, and harmful bacteria. Although the ratio of these three will differ from individual to individual, beneficial and intermediate bacteria account for most of the species, and some harmful species coexist with them.

Beneficial bacteria promote digestion, create nutrients, and suppress growth of harmful bacteria. They also suppress the formation of harmful substances, prevent absorption of harmful substances into the body by strengthening the intestinal wall, and help immune cells function normally, enabling them to eliminate mutated cells effectively. When the condition of the intestines is poor, harmful bacteria multiply excessively, which can cause inflammation, diarrhea, indigestion, constipation, hypertension, inhibited liver function, obesity, and inhibited anticancer capabilities. Intermediate bacteria

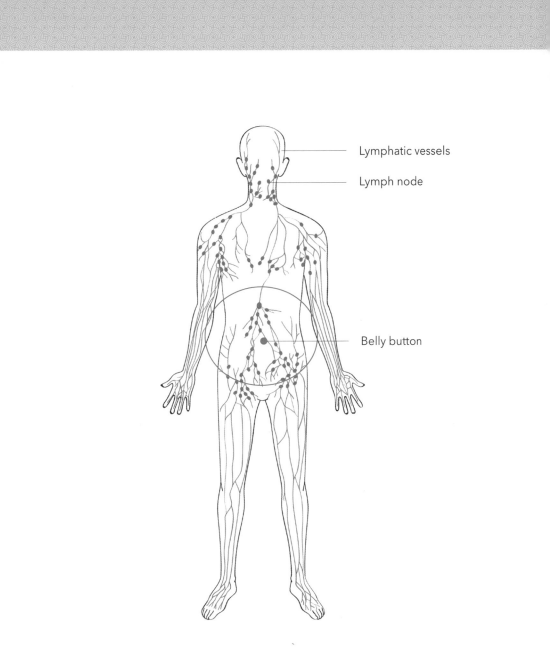

Lymphatic vessels

Lymph node

Belly button

THE LYMPHATIC SYSTEM AROUND YOUR BELLY BUTTON

differ in their roles depending on the gut environment. In other words, intermediate bacteria act as beneficial bacteria when the number of beneficial bacteria in the gut increases, then act as harmful bacteria when the number of harmful bacteria increases.

If you want to protect your intestinal health, it's important to increase the number of beneficial bacteria in your gut by improving its environment. "A person's death begins in the gut," said world-famous Russian biologist Ilya Ilyich Mechnikov. The enteric immune system, which includes the activity of immune cells and microbes in the gut, is essential, accounting for 70 to 80 percent of the whole body's immunity. That's how basic and central protecting the health of the intestines is to health in general.

It has been revealed through many clinical studies is that body temperature affects immune system function. Immune activity increases when body temperature rises within the normal range and decreases when it falls. Belly Button Healing helps you increase abdominal temperature by exercising and promoting blood circulation in the intestines, resulting in enhanced immunity.

Refresh and Vitalize Your Gut

You've heard over and over again that you need more exercise to be healthy. Yet, for most people, this simple piece of advice is so difficult to follow. Until just a few decades ago, people walked most places that they went and lived lives that involved a lot of physical activity. Lately, though, with the development of mechanized means of transportation, people move even short distances by car and sit in chairs, never taking their eyes off of their TV, smart phone, or computer screen. So there is no way they're going to walk much, unless they intentionally take the time for a walk, hike, or workout on a treadmill. Adding the effects of excessive stress, processed food, and environmental pollution makes it difficult for us to protect our intestinal health.

Our intestines, structurally, wind around in our abdominal cavity and have gaps between countless protruding villi, which provide plenty of space for food residue to stagnate. In particular, the toxins that are excreted when over-consumed animal proteins are broken down act as factors causing the intestines to stiffen. The intestines also become stiff when a state of stress-induced tension continues or when the left-right balance of the body is broken by bad posture. Saying that the intestines become "stiff" means that intestinal function is weakened by poor circulation and excretion, and that reduced intestinal motion leads to stagnation, which causes the formation and buildup of hard lumps. When you actually do Intestinal Massage, which will be introduced later, you'll find that the intestines of some people are soft while those of others are hard and don't give much.

If the intestines are stiff, resulting in an excessive discharge of active oxygen or toxins, this may put an increased burden on the liver to cleanse the body. The heart is also burdened more when blood circulation in the intestines slows. Toxins discharged in the intestines can accumulate in the synapses of the brain's neurons, causing problems in the transmission of nerve signals. This, in turn, can cause brain pathologies like cognitive and behavioral impairments, and can even lead to dementia. To prevent such problems, it's extremely important to create a healthy environment in the intestines.

Exercising the intestines is more effective than anything else for preventing or relieving stiffness. No one thinks they should consciously exercise their intestines, though, because they are not a part of the body we can touch directly or move how we want, like our arms and legs.

Also, stiffness and reduced intestinal function can lead to a situation in which putrefactive bacteria are always increasing in numbers when the balance in the intestines is broken. The role of putrefactive bacteria is breaking down the body of an organism. Putrefactive bacteria are not necessarily and only bad, but if their numbers grow too much, they can cause various diseases.

For example, when water is flowing well through a gorge, the microbes or minerals in it are in a state of optimum balance. The water putrefies and stinks, though, if its flow is blocked at some point. In other words, it now has too many putrefactive bacteria. Spraying a disinfectant because putrefactive bacteria have grown too numerous will kill the germs, but it could also cause a collapse in the natural ecosystem.

So the best way to solve the problem is to break through the blockages, enabling the water to flow naturally.

This also applies to the principles of Belly Button Healing. Through regular, rapid vibration and stimulation of the belly button, it exercises and relaxes stiff, less-active intestines and breaks through blockages, effectively restoring a natural, healthy intestinal ecosystem.

The more water putrefies, the more biological oxygen demand increases. When the concentration of organic matter in water increases, the activity and number of aerobic microorganisms that break down organic matter and purify the water also needs to increase. Microbial activity is inhibited by a lack of oxygen, however, so a regular oxygen supply is essential for purifying water. In the same way, a great deal of oxygen is required to discharge and purify toxins in our intestines as well as other areas of our bodies.

Belly Button Healing is a very effective method for increasing the amount of oxygen supplied to the body. When the intestines become more flexible through release of tension by Belly Button Healing, the diaphragm is able to move further into the abdominal cavity without extra effort. This increases the amount of air inhaled and therefore the amount of oxygen supplied to the body. The increased oxygen enables more vigorous purification of waste products and toxins from every nook and cranny of the intestines and the whole body, refreshing it and allowing it to recover vitality.

Unwind Your Entire Body

As the center of our bodies, the belly button also lies at the center of the body's extensive and continuous network of fascial tissue. This dense and strong yet flexible connective tissue made primarily of collagen can be described as a tightly-knit body suit that holds our organs in place, provides containers for our fat and inner fluids, and helps our bones and muscles keep their structure and move smoothly. Fascia covers and connects the entire body.

Normally, fascia is relaxed and can move without restriction. However, when it gets too tense due to factors such as maintaining one posture for a long time, repetitive movements such as typing, scarring from surgery, emotional or physical trauma, or inflammation, it becomes more difficult for our organs to function. Tense or restricted fascia can put pressure on the body and cause pain, stress, and limited motion as a result. Approximately 85 percent of visits to general practitioner physicians are a result of pain caused .

The pressing and massaging motions of Belly Button Healing release fascial tension. Because of the navel's location, pressing there relieves tension not only from the area around the belly button, but along the entire fascial network. It's one reason Belly Button Healing practitioners report greater relaxation, flexibility, and pain relief in areas from their pelvis, to their lower back, to their legs, arms, and necks. Along with the release of tension in the intestines and the abdominal muscles, release of tension in the fascia permits greater blood and lymph circulation throughout the body and food motility through the intestines.

From a physical perspective, Belly Button Healing, by stimulating the gut brain, increasing core temperature and blood circulation, enhancing the activity of gut microbes, and reducing fascial tension, helps improve our body's condition and natural healing capacity.

CHAPTER 3

The Energy Perspective

In order to understand Belly Button Healing from an energy perspective, I recommend that you first experience Belly Button Healing directly. Belly Button Healing is a very easy method, and you can feel its effects immediately. So, we'll try Belly Button Breathing now, which, as we'll see in Part 2, is Step 1 of Belly Button Healing.

First, lie comfortably on your back. A seated posture is also acceptable if you can't lie down at the moment. Comfortably relax your body and mind, and try to feel the condition of your body, such as your breathing rhythm, your sense of vitality, and the temperature of your belly and legs.

If you have a Belly Button Healing Wand, put the end of its longest section against your navel and press it repeatedly. Place it over your clothing, not on your bare skin. If you don't have a Belly Button Healing Wand, bring the tips of your index, middle, and ring fingers of both hands together and use them to press your navel repeatedly. Close your eyes and concentrate your awareness on your belly button, pressing it rhythmically as you do about 100 repetitions per minute.

If you have a constricted feeling in your chest at this time, exhale in sharp, short breaths through your nose or mouth, discharging the stagnant air and energy in your chest. Stop after about 100 repetitions. While in a comfortable posture, close your eyes and breathe, concentrating on your belly button and lower abdomen.

The basic process of Belly Button Healing is simple: repeatedly press your navel and then practice Belly Button Breathing after that. To maximize the effects of Belly Button Breathing, however, your imagination must be added to this exercise. Visualize that there is a breathing hole in your belly button, as if the nose on your face has moved to your navel.

Breathe in, push your belly out and visualize life energy entering and filling it through the "nose" of your navel, and, when you breathe out, concentrate your awareness in your navel as you cause your belly to contract, pulling it toward your back. Imagine that the energy of life is being injected into your abdomen through your navel as you visualize your belly repeatedly inflating and deflating like a rubber balloon. As you continue to breathe, check the following list to see what phenomena are occurring in your body.

1. Is your abdomen expanding and contracting naturally when you breathe?

2. Is your breathing going deeper, all the way into your abdomen?

3. Is your abdomen growing warmer?

4. Are your lower back and pelvis growing warmer?

5. Are your thighs, legs, and toes growing warmer?

6. Is a lot of saliva filling your mouth?

7. Is the tension in your body, including your neck and shoulders, being gradually released?

8. Is your head gradually becoming clearer?

9. Do you get the feeling that the blood circulation in your body is improving?

10. Overall, do you feel strength developing and vitality increasing in your body?

When you compare the state of your body now with its state before you did Belly Button Healing, how many of the ten items listed above did you feel?

If you felt seven or more, then you can accurately say that you are relatively healthy and that you have a keen energy sense. If you felt less than five, then your body may be tired or tense, and you may have a lot of thoughts, causing you to have trouble calling your consciousness into your body and focusing on physical sensations. In that case, you doing Belly Button Healing more frequently will help. If you press your navel again, about 100 more times, and, then, close your eyes and concentrate on the sensations in your body, you will feel them more clearly.

I believe that you probably felt at least five of the listed sensations. Think about it. With no more than about five minutes of Belly Button Breathing, your breathing deepened and became more natural, your abdomen and even your lower body grew warmer, your head became clearer, and you were charged with vital energy, while also becoming more relaxed. Isn't that amazing?

The Best Energy Point for Assisting Circulation

The key to Belly Button Healing is found in the position of the navel. The position of the belly button is truly marvelous when viewed from an energy perspective, as well as from a physical perspective.

Eastern medicine approaches the human body and conceives its principles of operation based on its understanding of vital energy, and, according to this system, our skin has holes through which energy enters and leaves our bodies. These are called meridian points or energy points, and they are used for healing. They may be stimulated with needles, moxibustion, or acupressure to improve the flow of energy.

In Eastern medicine, balanced and flowing energy is the

basis of good health. Our bodies have approximately 360 major energy points, many of which are concentrated in the head, hands, feet, and abdomen. The back side of your body collects Yang energy, which is hot and dry. The front side of your body collects Yin energy, which is cold and wet. If too much Yin energy collects in the abdomen, however, it creates imbalance and energy blockage, which leads to disease. To balance excessive Yin energy, Eastern medicine recommends warming the belly to add Yang energy.

Among the abdominal energy points that control Yin energy, an important one is found in the belly button. The Korean name of this navel energy point is *Shingwol*, or "palace of God," the place where God comes and goes and dwells. It is also called *Jejung*, which means "center of the body." Here, we can view God as signifying the very life energy of the cosmos. The belly button is a major energy point through which the life force enters our bodies.

The Shingwol is situated at the exact center of the belly button, and it is an important energy point used by traditional Asian doctors to control diseases that occur in the abdomen. According to Eastern medicine, stimulating the Shingwol point improves the body's immunity and facilitates the flow of energy and blood in the abdominal organs, while also warming the body and restoring its overall health.

The Shingwol point is closely associated with the small and large intestines, which, as you know, are in charge of converting food into nutrients through the process of digestion.

These nutrients react with the oxygen and energy obtained through respiration to become the vital energy of our bodies.

If you experienced your belly naturally expanding and contracting more deeply when you did Belly Button Breathing a moment ago, it means that the Shingwol in your belly button was activated and that energy is entering it well. As you practice this, it's important to feel and visualize the energy of life entering the belly button.

On the human body, the Shingwol functions like the roots of a tree. When a tree's roots are supplied with nutrients, its branches and leaves grow rich and luxurious, its flowers bloom, and it bears good fruit. The Shingwol's role is similar, since it is the place where we received energy and blood from our mothers when we were in her womb. Thus, through focused Belly Button Breathing, we are, in essence, supplied with energy through the root of our bodies. Our bodies are filled with vital energy, and our immune and circulatory systems are stimulated, which may prevent or heal various diseases.

Just as there are channels in our bodies through which blood and lymphatic fluid flow, there are also pathways along which energy flows. These are called "meridians," and major energy points are located along them. The major meridians are the twelve meridians that are associated with twelve of the body's organs. For Belly Button Healing, there are two additional meridians that are especially important: the Conception Meridian, which is located on a central line at the front of the upper body, and the Governor Meridian, which is on a central line at the back of the body. The belly button and the Shingwol point are located on the Conception Meridian.

When you tried Belly Button Breathing a moment ago, did you feel your lower back, pelvis, abdomen, and lower body growing warmer? More than likely, you did, because, by pressing your Shingwol, you activated the flow of energy along your Conception and Governor meridians. These two meridians flow into each other, creating a circle along a central line at the front and back of your trunk. When you press your belly button, energy activated in the Shingwol flows down along your Conception Meridian, passes your lower abdomen and pelvis, and flows into the Governor Meridian at the back of your trunk. Then, it circulates along your Governor Meridian up to your lower back and spine.

Did you also feel your lower back warming when you did Belly Button Breathing? The reason is that the energy along your back in your Governor Meridian was activated. People with an especially well-developed energy sense clearly feel the activation of energy here when they do Belly Button Breathing. In that area, the *Myungmoon* point, is located opposite your belly button. Situated on your Governor Meridian, it is an energy point at a spot intersected by a horizontal line drawn from your belly button to your spine. Myungmoon means "the gate that life enters." When the flow of energy is activated in this spot, life energy can be felt passing through it into the abdomen. The Shingwol and Myungmoon are major energy points for activating the *Dahnjon* system, which will

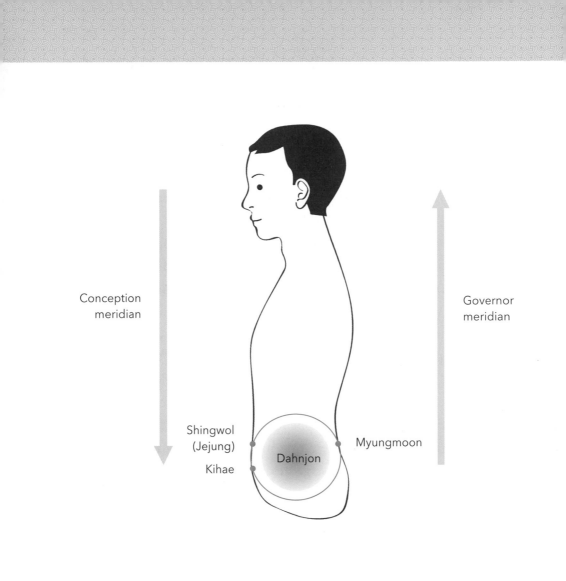

Conception
meridian

Governor
meridian

Shingwol
(Jejung)

Kihae

Dahnjon

Myungmoon

IMPORTANT ENERGY POINTS AND CHANNELS
AROUND THE BELLY BUTTON

be described later. When these energy points are activated, you will feel your abdomen growing warmer, along with your breathing growing deeper.

When the abdomen is heated, that warm energy pushes the water energy of the kidneys up toward the head. Rising along the Governor Meridian, the water energy cools the fire energy in the head and heart. That's why, if you do Belly Button Breathing for a while, you'll find your abdomen and lower body growing warmer, but your head becoming clearer, your shoulders and neck relaxing, and sweet saliva filling your mouth. In short, you will feel a warm belly and a cool head. This phenomenon is called *Suseung Hwagang*, or "Water Up, Fire Down," the properly balanced and healthy flow of energy in your body. If the rhythm of this energy circulation is disrupted, the opposite phenomenon develops: fire energy stagnates in the head, resulting in headaches and insomnia, and cold water energy stagnates in the abdomen, resulting in problems with digestive function and with energy and blood circulation.

Water Up, Fire Down develops when energy circulates normally along the circle created by the Conception and Governor meridians. People who do energy training know that it's very important to activate these two meridians. This is because the 12 meridians are also activated in a chain reaction when the Conception and Governor meridians are activated. Half of the 12 meridians are Yin meridians and the other half are Yang meridians. The six Yin meridians are controlled by the Conception Meridian, and the remaining six Yang meridians are controlled by the Governor Meridian. Consequently, circulating energy through the Conception and Governor meridians is directly connected with activation of the 12 meridians, and, furthermore, with circulation of energy throughout the body.

The belly button is the best acupressure point, and Belly Button Healing is the simplest and most effective method for activating Water Up, Fire Down, the normal and balanced state of energy circulation in the human body.

The Activation Button for Deep Energy Breathing

It's easy for people to think that the lungs themselves do the breathing, because air enters and leaves them when we breathe. The lungs have no muscles, however, so they cannot breathe on their own.

The movements of the thoracic muscles and the diaphragm make it possible for the lungs to breathe. When you inhale, your chest expands and your diaphragm sinks downward. The diaphragm is a muscular membrane situated horizontally between the lungs and the abdomen. When its muscles move downward, the space in the chest cavity expands, which lowers its internal air pressure. Outside air naturally enters the lungs as a result of this pressure difference. The movement of the diaphragm plays such an important role in determining lung capacity that the lungs take in 250 to 300 cubic centimeters more air when the diaphragm moves downward just a centimeter.

You may have heard the terms chest breathing and abdominal breathing. Chest breathing is a kind of shallow respiration that is generally driven by the movements of the thoracic muscles. It is seen a lot in women or in people whose torso is tense. Abdominal breathing, on the other hand, is driven by the movement of the diaphragm. It allows for deeper and slower respiration than chest breathing, and it is generally seen a lot in males and infants.

There is a strong association between the length of our breaths and the health of our bodies and minds. We do abdominal breathing when we are young and healthy, until, as we get older and our bodies become weaker, our breathing gradually becomes shorter and shallower. Normally, the length of a breath is four to five seconds. When we're under stress or moving vigorously, this shortens to one to two seconds. The tortoise, which is well-known for its long lifespan of up to 300 years, is said to take 20 to 30 seconds for a single breath. This fact shows how much slow, deep breathing contributes to health and longevity.

In addition to diaphragm movement, there is another important element in abdominal breathing. It's the movement of the abdominal muscles. Abdominal pressure forms when the diaphragm moves into the abdomen during inhalation, which naturally causes the belly to expand outward. Breathing slowly and deeply using the movement of the abdominal muscles is not only effective for promoting blood circulation and relieving stress, but it is also extremely effective for increasing lung capacity. That's why people who sing or play a musical instrument train in this type of abdominal breathing.

For many years, I have taught methods of breathing based on Korea's traditional mind-body training method, *Sundo*. It couples energy sensitivity with abdominal breathing, and it is called Dahnjon Breathing. It moves the diaphragm and abdominal muscles as is done in abdominal breathing, but it also includes breathing that follows the sensation of energy in the abdomen.

The word Dahnjon refers to an energy center where vital energy accumulates. In Dahnjon Breathing, the most important energy center is located in the middle of the lower abdomen at a *Kihae* point about two inches below the navel and two inches inside the body. The purpose of Dahnjon Breathing is to activate this energy core, to warm the abdomen, and to circulate vital energy throughout the body.

Dahnjon Breathing is centered on the Dahnjon, and it activates the major energy points around it. The points are the Shingwol in the navel, the Kihae, two inches below the navel, and the Myungmoon, situated at the back, opposite the navel. Altogether, they are called the Dahnjon System.

As you do Dahnjon Breathing, it is important to sense the energy of the Dahnjon System. Immediately feeling energy is not easy for people who have never done energy training or who are beginners. Even those who have done some training may miss the sense of the Dahnjon if they lack physical vitality or sufficient concentration. Dahnjon Breathing activates the energy of the core through concentrated awareness, like blowing on a fire with a bellows, and it circulates energy to the whole body. This may take a long time for those whose core energy is weak. If a fire is already burning, it's easy to make it blaze by blowing on it, but a fire must be rekindled if it has gone out.

I have discovered, though, that, through just five minutes of Belly Button Breathing, you can feel energy in your body that you would normally only sense after 30 minutes of Dahnjon Breathing. So, I am hopeful that Belly Button Breathing will give even greater help to more people, especially those whose basic physical condition is poor.

If you breathe comfortably after repeatedly pressing your belly button, your lower abdomen immediately becomes warmer, as if you had kindled a fire in it, and your Dahnjon System starts to operate so that more energy gathers and circulates throughout your body. As it does, you can feel your lower body growing warmer, all the way to your toes. Your blood circulation also increases, adding to this effect.

Another advantage of Belly Button Healing is that after doing it, you don't need to push out and pull in your abdomen consciously as you do with Dahnjon Breathing alone. Because Belly Button Healing relaxes your abdomen, your abdomen moves in and out effortlessly and deeply, turning your breathing into Dahnjon Breathing naturally.

Breathe for a while, imagining that life energy is entering through your navel. The Myungmoon point at your back will open further, bringing in more energy, which will instantly circulate in your Dahnjon. If you focus on this energy sense, enough pressure will form in your abdomen so that you will feel a force naturally supporting your body's core.

Soon you will experience for yourself that the navel is the best button for activating deep energy breathing.

Belly Button Healing, Energy CPR

In Eastern medicine, the Shingwol energy point is used for emergency treatment when a person has suddenly lost consciousness or has collapsed due to high blood pressure or stroke. It is also applied when treating intestinal diseases that come from low body temperature, cold limbs, or women's reproductive issues, such as menstrual disorders and infertility.

I've witnessed that many people experience their bodies growing warmer and their breathing growing deeper and more stable after their energy and blood circulation improved after doing Belly Button Healing. It has occurred to me that Belly Button Healing is a kind of first aid for people whose vitality has declined. It's similar to how we use CPR on someone whose heart has stopped. Belly Button Healing, we could say, is energy CPR for reviving the vitality of someone whose health has collapsed.

There is a fascinating study by a research team from Patterson Medical Center and Joseph Medical Group that provided treatment for resuscitating 103 emergency patients whose breathing was gradually stopping. There were two kinds of treatment: one was the conventional method of doing only chest compressions; the other was a method that involved alternating chest and abdominal compressions. Amazingly, the recovery rate with the chest-compression method was no more than seven percent, but the recovery rate with the alternating chest and abdominal compression method reached a surprising 25 percent.

By compressing the abdomen, it is possible to pump blood collecting in the intestines, circulating it throughout the body. This movement also exercises the abdominal muscles and makes the intestines flexible, allowing the diaphragm to sink deeply into the abdomen. So, when you lack vitality or you're tired, if you press your belly button, even for a moment, and then do Belly Button Breathing, you will soon feel your body recovering vigor and growing warmer.

You can identify the state of the person's health just by checking whether their abdomen is warm or cold, soft or hard. People who lack vitality and who have health problems often have cold bellies and stiff intestines. If your body temperature usually falls to below 96.8 degrees Fahrenheit (36 degrees Celsius), it is an ominous danger sign for your health.

When your body temperature is low, your blood circulation, metabolism, and detoxification functions are weakened and your immunity is lowered. You also easily gain abdominal fat when your belly is cold. This is because waste products are not readily processed under such conditions, creating an environment in which fat easily accumulates. Consequently, if you keep your belly warm, you can more easily lose weight.

Although raising body temperature through exercise is a good approach, in people whose level of basic fitness is low, body temperature can drop after exercising for some time, and exercising too much consumes basic energy, which could have the opposite effect. So, people need to exercise in a way that's right for their own condition. The goal is to promote good energy and blood circulation throughout the day through a consistent practice of deep breathing.

To increase body temperature, it's important to warm the abdomen, which is the body's core. Breathing must deepen if the abdomen is to become warmer. When you do deep breathing, your diaphragm sinks farther into your abdomen, pressing against your abdominal organs. In effect, this massages the organs and promotes blood circulation. Belly Button Healing naturally induces deep breathing, which not only makes the abdomen warmer, but also causes that warmth to spread throughout the body, all the way to the fingers and toes, so it is excellent for recovering full-body vitality.

Scattered thoughts and a consciousness directed outward are often the root cause of poor fitness and shallow breathing. One method of energy training is concentrating awareness on the Dahnjon System in the lower abdomen to quiet thoughts and to bring consciousness back into the body. If you breathe for a while, concentrating your mind in your Dahnjon and belly button, vital energy will build up in your core, your breathing will automatically stabilize and grow deeper, and your mind will become stable and centered.

How Should You Care for Your Belly Button?

You may have noticed that material readily accumulates in the folds of your belly button. This is usually a buildup of fibers or cellular debris, along with various microbial organisms. Although the number and types of microbes differ from person to person, according to a 2012 study by North Carolina State University, approximately 70 different species live in the belly button.

The researchers said, "Thousands of bacteria live in our navels, like a rain forest. It's quite beautiful." Most of the microbes living on our skin, including those in our navel, not only cause no harm to their host, but they even act as a defense force, protecting the skin from harmful bacteria.

So, aside from taking regular baths or showers, you don't need to clean your belly button much, especially because it contains a team of very helpful bacteria. If you try to forcibly extract the debris stuck in your belly button, you could cause injury or get an infection because the skin tissue of your navel is weak. Just gently wipe away only the visible areas with a cotton swab.

For cleanliness and not to irritate this area when you do Belly Button Healing, it's better to place your fingers over your clothing or a towel, not on your bare skin.

CHAPTER 4

The Philosophical Perspective

At first, my interest in the belly button was strictly practical. I saw it as a possible method for healing the body and stabilizing the mind. The more I became familiar with the navel, though, the deeper its significance grew for me, and, as I did deep Belly Button Breathing, I had an incredibly profound realization concerning the nature of life.

As I practiced it more, I could feel life energy entering my body through my belly button, and as my breathing grew deeper and more comfortable, I returned to my mother's womb and felt a supply of life energy moving through my umbilical cord. It was as if I was going back to that infinitely comfortable and peaceful time, when I was receiving the love of my mother in that safe, cozy place. Instead of feeling like I was a separate organism, I had a sense of stability and unity, of being connected with my mother through my belly button.

My mother was also connected through her umbilical cord to her mother. If we follow the ancestral line of our umbilical cord from our mother, to her mother's mother, her mother's mother's mother, and so on, eventually we will reach our primal mother—the one we all share. The umbilical cord is a precious lifeline that began in my primal mother and has come down to me. My belly button is undeniable, visual proof that I'm not a separate organism, but that I am connected with the Source of life.

A Seal from the Source of Life

For me, my belly button is not simply a trace of my birth, but a precious seal and a mark, a reminder of my connection with the Source of life and all life forms. Our bodies live separately from each other, but we are deeply connected with each other, through our belly buttons, to the Source of life.

Every time I feel my belly button, I feel great gratitude that I have a navel. I'm grateful to be alive, I'm grateful that I'm connected with the incredible life force of the universe, and I am overwhelmed with gratitude that I am receiving the blessings of life energy. The gratitude and humbleness I feel before the great cycle of life automatically fills my heart to overflowing.

Everyone in this world has a navel. We all grew in our mother's womb, thanks to a supply of nutrients received through our umbilical cords, and then we were born into this world. Though our skin colors may be different, though our languages may be different, as we look at the belly button, the symbol of our ultimate connection, we should remember that we are one family that has come from the same Source of life.

Activate Your Natural Intelligence

No one can live your life for you. It is you—and no one else—who assigns meaning and value to your individual life. For that reason, you have very important decisions to make. What will you value most in your life? And what goals will you pursue? It is easy to let others influence you when you decide the answers to these questions, but only you can make appropriate decisions about them.

Your life is like a voyage taken in a great ocean vessel, and you are the captain of that ship. To take yourself where you want to go in life, you must have your hands on the steering wheel at all times, directing the rudder appropriately. We all know this well enough, yet living accordingly is not always easy. Too often, we are swept away by our environment. Family members demand that obligations be met, and financial realities keep us tied down and overly busy. Other times, the opinions of others convince us to ignore the voice we hear inside, or information from society at large tricks us into believing that our highest goals are impossible or even dangerous.

But there is an important thing to remember: you cannot discover your true worth through information. The ideas and emotions that keep you from your highest self are nothing more than that—information. Just because you read a lot of books and graduated from a good college, just because you have wealth and power, just because you've grown older does not mean that you will discover your true value and the real purpose of your life.

The knowledge we acquire in school and the information we obtain from the world, although useful at times, is mostly artificial, surface-level knowledge. A truthful, authentic life comes to us through realizations that happen within us, not through the gathering of worldly knowledge. When we seek knowledge from deep inside, our true consciousness and the ability to gain mastery over our lives awakens. I call this consciousness "natural intelligence" because it is something that always exists within us, awaiting activation. The key to awakening this natural intelligence is to encounter the life force within you. Your true identity is the indwelling life force within you, and it is naturalness itself—existing beyond artificial knowledge or information. The true central value of your life may only be found there.

For many years, I have worked to develop better methods of uncovering this value, but Belly Button Healing is the simplest and most effective method I have come across yet. As countless people are discovering for themselves, Belly Button Healing produces amazing and diverse benefits: improved energy and blood circulation, promotion of hormone secretion through stimulation of the enteric nervous system, relief of chronic pain, deep and stable breathing, enhanced immunity, increased concentration and creativity, and weight loss.

People who have reconnected with their life force know that they are nature itself and that they have found their true value. Such people listen to the inner voice of their true nature instead of the voice of knowledge, ideas, and emotions. This inner voice is our natural intelligence, an intelligence that manifests from the center of life itself. When this ability begins to operate, you will become a true creator of your life.

People who have awakened their natural intelligence always keep their hands on the steering wheel of life; they are never swept away by the flow of life. They're people who sail forward with a firm grip on the wheel, directing the ship of their lives. They choose to do good for themselves, for others, and for the world with a sense of direction and centeredness rooted in their natural intelligence. Such people are needed in these times.

Connecting to your life force is the truest and most powerful way to begin the process of growth and change. I discovered this secret in the belly button, the very center of our bodies. Belly Button Healing is an amazing tool that starts you on the path toward healing body and mind, developing infinite creativity, and healing the world and the earth.

From the Belly Button to the Earth

One of the greatest joys that I have had while teaching Belly Button Healing is seeing people start expanding their awareness from their belly button to the Earth. "From the belly button to the Earth?" You may question the meaning of these words or think this is too great a leap.

However, if you open yourself to feeling a connection to something bigger than yourself through Belly Button Healing, I believe you, too, will feel the same way other practitioners have. Just as you can feel connected to your line of human mothers through your belly button, you can feel an ultimate connection to the Earth mother on whom all of our lives depend.

As you do Belly Button Healing, you develop a sense of familiarity and friendliness with yourself, and you manifest a bond of empathy with yourself. When this happens, you deepen your sensibility and become more aware of your thoughts, emotions, words, and habits. This naturally motivates you to make positive changes in your life.

The growing empathy you experience through Belly Button Healing doesn't just stay inside you. It spreads out to all of the relationships you have—to your family, your friends, the communities you belong to, and ultimately to our greater home, planet Earth. In the same way that greater empathy motivates you to change yourself, as your empathy encapsulates the planet, you become motivated to make a positive impact on the world.

I urge you to clearly understand this simple truth: Everything ultimately starts inside you. First, you must become one with yourself and have an inner awakening. Then, you can feel your connection with the Source of life through a simple touch of your belly button. Similarly, if you are connected and one with yourself, even something as massive as the Earth feels as if it belongs to you, something you want to love and care for.

As I explained earlier, the microbes in your gut play an important role in your immune system. They are also essential in digestion, vitamin production, and mood regulation. Microbes are not only present in the digestive tract, but can be found on your skin, including in the navel itself, and numerous other places. In the human body, there are 10 times more microbes than human cells—10 trillion human cells and 100 trillion microbes. So, we carry around bodies that are 10 percent human and 90 percent microbial. Meanwhile, the total weight of those microbes is only one to three percent of our body weight.

The antibiotics that many people take to kill bacteria that are harming them, however, also kill even the beneficial bacteria in our bodies. Using an antibiotic to kill several types of targeted bacteria is the same as burning down a house to kill a few fleas inside. We must remember that our body is an ecosystem. This ecosystem must be maintained, and our immunity strengthened, by caring for the small organisms inside us, instead of by killing them haphazardly with harmful drugs or foods. Our body teaches us that health lies in balance and harmony, rather than in conflict and fighting.

It's important to go a step further: to care for organisms

outside our bodies just as we care for the organisms inside it. The earth herself is an organism in her own right, and she needs our care, too. It will be impossible for us to maintain the health of the organism called the earth unless we feel and care for other organisms as we do for ourselves—and unless we take action. Killing all the microbes—including beneficial ones—in our bodies with antibiotics and causing harm to others or the environment for our own benefit reflects the same self-centered attitude that has produced our current environmental emergency. Ultimately, our individual state of health will not be maintained if the ecosystem in our bodies breaks down.

Protecting the health of your gut and protecting the external ecosystem are both about caring for and protecting life. If the desire to care for our own health through Belly Button Healing spreads, it will connect with each person's natural aspiration to protect other lifeforms on the earth. Thus, your desire to care for the condition of your gut is an attitude that, ultimately, can save the planet.

The distance from your belly button to the earth is not long. Through our belly buttons, not only can we connect with ourselves, but we also gain the wisdom to see the earth as an extension of ourselves. Through Belly Button Healing, we can nurture a mindset that can heal us as individuals and the entire planet as a whole.

This is a core message I've been sharing since I began teaching natural healing methods to people in a Korean park in 1980. Now, more than 35 years later, these aspirations have come together to form a global endeavor called the Earth Citizen Movement.

Earth Citizens are people who care for the earth as they care for their own bodies. They have minds and hearts that know the Earth is the foundation of everything they do. They recognize themselves as members of a planetary community, instead of as members of a single nation, religion, or organization. And, most importantly, they live that awareness.

Becoming an Earth Citizen begins in your heart. Every time you see your belly button, remember that your life is connected with the life of the planet, and, every time you do Belly Button Healing, remember that you can also care for the earth's life forms the way you care for the many organisms coexisting in your body.

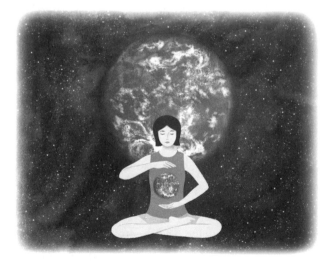

You always carry your belly button around with you. Your belly button is truly a connection point to yourself, other people, other life forms, and our planet earth.

Whenever you do Belly Button Healing for yourself or for others, please do so with this awareness, and let the awareness spread into every aspect of your life. In a sense, you, I, and each one of us form the belly button of the human family. You are an indispensable and irreplaceable asset to this family. Whatever you do, big or small, it ultimately affects all life on earth.

I offer my humble admiration for your beautiful heart that seeks to help others live a healthy, happy, and meaningful life. I hope my Belly Button Healing method can assist you in manifesting a more caring heart toward yourself and others.

12 Benefits of Belly Button Healing

1. Promotes blood circulation

Belly Button Healing promotes blood circulation by stimulating the abdominal organs, which contain about 30 to 40 percent of the body's blood volume. It also assists circulation in the abdominal aorta and inferior vena cava, which are behind the belly button. The repeated movements warm the abdomen, inducing the blood vessels to dilate, which allows more blood to flow through them.

Furthermore, pressing and massaging your calves and the soles of your feet using the Belly Button Healing Wand also greatly helps with blood circulation. The calves and soles of the feet play such an important role in blood circulation that they are called "the second heart."

2. Warms abdomen, increases body temperature

You can immediately feel your lower body, from your abdomen all the way to your toes, growing warmer when you do Belly Button Healing, thanks to improved energy and blood circulation. Rising body temperature improves your metabolism and your immune and detoxification functions.

3. Improves digestive and excretory functions

The enteric nervous system spread out in the abdomen is stimulated, promoting intestinal peristalsis and churning, which results in good digestion and smooth bowel activity.

4. Relieves pain and tension in joints

The abdomen is connected to joints in your pelvis, legs, and arms through fascia and blood vessels. Tension in the fascia and muscles is released, which allows the body to realign itself better, improving overall flexibility and relieving pain from improper posture.

5. Increases immunity and detoxification

Lymph nodes concentrated around the navel are stimulated, resulting in improved circulation of lymphatic fluid, which is involved in immunity and the excretion of waste and toxins. Also, the intestinal ecosystem becomes healthier, and these effects are further amplified with the resulting increased activity among enteric immune cells and microbes.

6. Augments physical vitality

The supply of oxygen and nutrients to the whole body is improved with blood circulation and deep breathing, and vital energy in the abdomen, the body's core, circulates throughout the body, increasing its vitality.

7. Clears head and improves concentration

Blood circulation and deep breathing supply plenty of oxygen to the brain, and the water energy of the kidneys rises to the head and cools the hot energy there, bringing greater mental clarity and better vision.

8. Relaxes body and mind

Concentrating on the outgoing breath during Belly Button Healing develops a state of parasympathetic dominance. The "rest and digest" state this creates relaxes the body, charges it with energy, and repairs its damaged areas.

9. Expands physical and mental well-being

Serotonin, 90 percent of which is secreted in the gut, improves our mood and gives us a feeling of well-being. Depression and anxiety, which appear when we don't have enough serotonin, may be problems of the gut, not the brain. Stimulation of the enteric nervous system increases our feelings of well-being, satisfaction, and ambition.

10. Makes skin lustrous and smooth

Improvement of general circulatory functions, such as those of the blood system, lymphatic system, nervous system, and digestive system, as well as of immune, digestive, and excretory functions, facilitates excretion of waste products and toxins. Improvement in the excretory functions of the whole body reduces the burden on the skin, which serves as an excretory organ, making it cleaner and more lustrous.

11. Strengthens familial bonds of love

Belly Button Healing allows you to care for the health of your family as well as your own health. As they perform Belly Button Healing on each other and talk about its effects, your family will more naturally feel and express deeper bonds and closeness.

12. Creates feelings of centeredness

Breathing while focusing on your navel brings your scattered mind back inside of your body, making you feel centered.

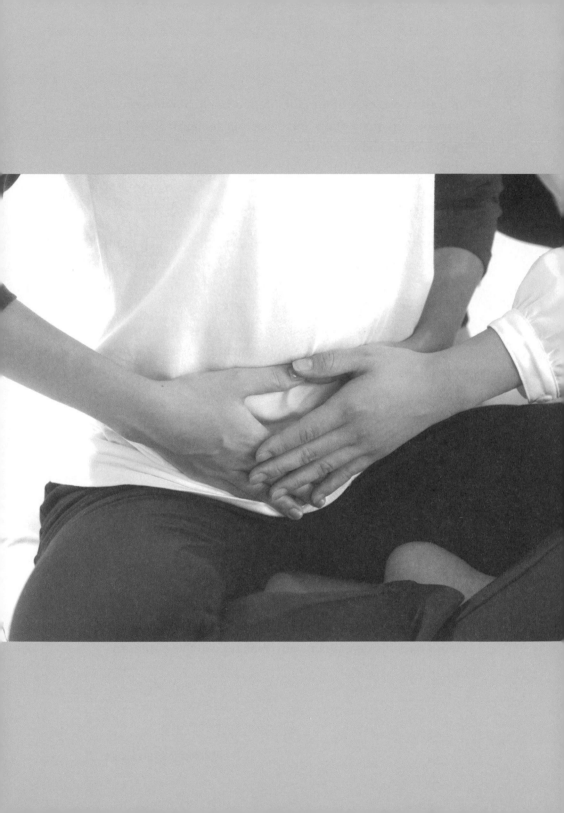

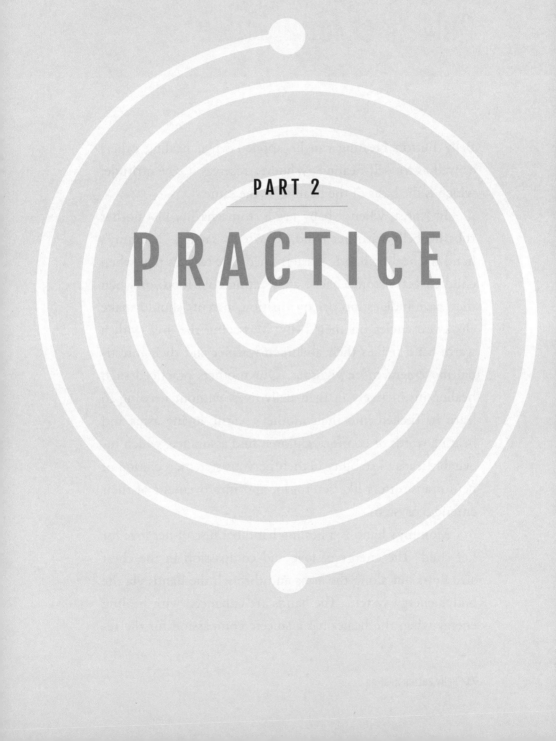

PART 2

PRACTICE

CHAPTER 5
Guidelines for Practice

Belly Button Healing can be applied when healing others as well as for self-healing. Whoever receives it, the attitude, which is the basis of the healing, is the same.

In Korea, when a baby has a stomachache, his mother rubs his belly with her hand, repeatedly saying, "Mommy's hand is a healing hand." Eastern medicine teaches that when children get a stomachache after eating cold food, or when they have indigestion or constipation, parents should make clockwise circles on their belly. Massaging the area with a warm hand makes their abdomen warmer and their intestinal movement more vigorous. Our mothers practiced such healing instinctively in their daily lives, without needing to learn it. Tucked into their mother's warm, loving arms and hearing words of comfort, children find assurance, which inevitably leads to stability in their nervous system, secretion of neurotransmitters like serotonin, and improvement of their enteric ecosystem.

Mommy's hand is a healing hand because of her love for her child. The energy of love and compassion in the chest area flows out along the arms and through the hands via the body's energy system. The hands are enhanced with healing energy when the healer has a sincere compassion for the receiver, a desire for their quick recovery, and a sincere wish for their improved health. Even when you heal yourself, if you press and massage your body with a caring heart and with gratitude for how precious it is, your body responds to that energy of love. Love is medicine. Love makes healing hands, and love increases the body's self-healing capacity.

Some studies have indicated that even just holding the hand of someone you love actually reduces stress and pain. This is because secretion of the stress hormone cortisol decreases while secretion of oxytocin, which is called the "cuddle hormone" or the "love hormone," increases, bringing feelings of psychological security and trust.

Renowned English animal behaviorist Desmond Morris says that animal grooming behavior, which prevents infections, developed in humans as a way for them to strengthen feelings of closeness and bonds of affection while caring for each other's bodies. Belly Button Healing, which anyone can do easily, is a great way to strengthen closeness and affection, especially among family members.

Your Body Is Nature

In addition to love, which is the first, most basic attitude for healing, there is an important second attitude. It's realizing that the body is a natural organism and believing in its natural healing power.

Our bodies react when they receive healing because they are natural. The body is not just a piece of wood or an inanimate lump of flesh. It is an organic life form in which the life energy of nature is condensed and circulates following the principles of energy. For example, if you press and massage places where energy is blocked, the blockages are released, and the energy starts to circulate again vigorously. Also, when fire energy collects in your head and causes a headache, if you apply healing techniques that expel excess fire energy and release the tension blocking it, the fire energy will sink into the abdomen. Then, you'll be able to recover your natural state of energy circulation, in which your belly is warm and your head cool.

When our health has deteriorated, passively accepting drugs or medical treatment is not our only option for recovery. We can also manifest the body's natural healing power, which assists it in returning to its original, healthy condition, through appropriate exercise, diet, and the use of natural health remedies. The body is natural, not mechanical. Our bodies have a natural restorative power that is not completely quantifiable, but it is real.

We should help our bodies manifest and maximize their

amazing life force. For this, we should minimize or eliminate those elements of our lifestyles that get in the way, and we should enhance and increase those elements that contribute to it. When we fully understand that our bodies are living, organic things, we develop a sensitivity for managing them. Without a close connection to our bodies, we may abuse them without even realizing it. Casually eating harmful foods, overeating, bad diets, drinking alcohol, smoking, overwork, stress, bad posture, bad life habits—all of these things are abuses we inflict on our bodies.

To prevent this, we should begin by listening to and taking an interest in the feelings of our bodies. If we focus on our bodies carefully, we can feel what foods and habits are bad for us and make our bodies uncomfortable. Then, if we examine the underlying reasons that we make poor choices, we will gradually be able to make better choices.

Belly Button Healing is an ongoing process of getting to know our bodies. Through it, we realize that a loving, caring heart is the fundamental power of healing and that everyone has healing energy and power. Also, we grow to believe in the wondrous abilities already built into our bodies and to know that all we need to do is awaken these abilities.

The greatest thing about Belly Button Healing is that we don't necessarily have to devote a lot of time to learning how to do it and to perfecting the techniques. Just apply it. That is all anyone has to do. Although we have a specialized tool for performing Belly Button Healing more easily and efficiently, if you don't have one immediately available, just use your hands. You could also apply another tool that functions like the specialized tool.

Healing happens naturally, and our sense of healing develops as we concentrate on our bodies and attentively examine their reactions.

Adopt a Healing Attitude

In order to use Belly Button Healing to maximize your body's natural healing power, maintain the following basic mindset.

- Release tension of body and mind. Healing is about causing the body to return to its natural state, so comfortably calming the mind comes before anything else when we perform healing, whether it's on ourselves or another person.

- Healing energy is shared by the people giving and receiving the healing. Waves of healing energy are amplified when the person performing the healing does so with a desire for the health and happiness of the receiver, and when the person receiving the healing approaches it with a grateful heart.

- If a person complains of pain when your hand barely touches their belly button, psychological tension rather than a physical problem could be the cause. You first need to explore other methods for releasing the tension, such as rubbing the abdomen with your palms or gently pressing and shaking the abdomen. Then, with attentive care, gradually apply Belly Button Healing after the person is relaxed.

Main Belly Button Healing Techniques

There are two main techniques that comprise Belly Button Healing. They are divided into two steps:

- **Step 1: Belly Button Breathing** is for promoting energy and blood circulation in the body by rhythmically and repeatedly pressing the navel.

- **Step 2: Belly Button Massage** is for finding pain points in the navel and its surrounding area and for resolving problems in associated parts of the body using massage.

These two techniques can be used separately from each other in any order, and auxiliary exercises, which will be described later, can be added to them.

Points to Keep in Mind Before Doing Belly Button Healing

1. You can do Belly Button Healing at any time, but it's best to avoid doing it immediately after a meal.

2. Before doing Belly Button Healing with your hands, make sure that your hands and nails are clean, and that your fingernails are short and smooth enough that they will not harm you or the person you will give a healing to.

3. Use Healing Life—the Belly Button Healing Wand—primarily on yourself. When you do use it to perform Belly Button Healing on another person, use the tool carefully and only after fully developing a sense for it by first using it on your own body.

4. Children seven years old and younger should not do Belly Button Healing using a tool because their intestines are weak. When a child has a stomachache or a cold, or is in poor physical condition, it's okay to gently massage the child's belly using the palm of your hand. Sweep down, gently rub, or slightly shake their belly, always keeping it warm.

5. Do not perform Belly Button Healing on pregnant women, patients with medical conditions, the infirm, people

with intestinal problems, people with weak vascular systems, people who have had abdominal surgery and have not yet healed, or those who have injuries near their navel.

6. Be careful not to apply too much pressure when using a Belly Button Healing Wand on the elderly, because their abdominal skin and intestines are weak. Whenever you do use the wand, carefully examine the health of the receiver to determine the appropriate intensity and speed.

7. You shouldn't press too forcefully on the navel of anyone who has high blood pressure, heart disease, or hardening of the abdominal arteries. It is especially important to avoid applying pressure too deeply to the left of the navel, where the aorta passes. Too much pressure could result in a sudden jump in blood pressure or in damage to the aorta. Gentle pressure is enough to have a beneficial result from Belly Button Healing.

8. Areas where the receiver feels pain when pressed should be handled very cautiously. Just pressing forcefully or for a long time does not make the pain go away. It's good

to approach a pain point gradually as you relax the area around it before pressing the point directly. Gently press on the pain point and relax it using massage or gentle vibration.

9. When using the Belly Button Healing Wand, it's safe to apply the device over the clothes, not on bare skin. Applying it directly to skin may cause irritation and reddening. If the receiver has very little abdominal fat and thin skin, first place a towel over her clothes before doing Belly Button Healing.

10. After practicing Belly Button Healing, especially after Belly Button Massage, pain or swelling could remain in the area where stimulation was focused. If that happens, instead of doing Belly Button Healing immediately the next day, take a break for a few days and then resume the practice after the pain disappears.

11. You can perform Belly Button Healing using another tool besides the Belly Button Healing Wand. If you do, carefully examine the form and material of the device, being sure to choose something appropriate. You shouldn't use something pointed, and avoid anything made of material that bends or breaks easily. And, of course, the hand is a suitable tool for Belly Button Healing. When using your hand, you can feel your body's warmth directly and can apply its use with greater sensitivity than you might with some other object.

When Is It Good to Do Belly Button Healing?

Belly Button Healing is such a quick and easy health practice that you can do it anytime during the day. It is especially helpful for managing your health if you apply it in the following circumstances:

- After you wake up, while you're still lying down
- Before getting up after you've taken a break
- When you feel weak or tired and need vitality
- When you want to calm your mind
- When you need focus
- When your body is tense
- When you feel bloated, or have diarrhea or constipation
- When your hands and feet are cold or you feel a chill
- When you need to relax your body and mind before going to sleep

The benefits of this practice will be doubled if, afterward, you do Intestinal Exercise or Intestinal Massage, which will be introduced later. Also, after practice, put your hands on your abdomen and breathe deeply, sending warm energy to your belly.

What Is a Belly Button Healing Wand?

While pressing on the belly button, it can be difficult to continue applying pressure with your hand. The Belly Button Healing Wand was created to make the practice easier. Called "Healing Life," this tool is shaped like a T, so it can be employed from a comfortable position without causing undue tension in the shoulders and chest.

The Belly Button Healing Wand has four points of application. By length, the longest is Inbong (literally, "human staff"), and the next are Jibong ("earth staff") and Chunbong ("heaven staff") respectively. The small knob is an acupressure knob. Usually Inbong is used for Belly Button Healing. If you want more gentle healing, you can use the thicker ends, Jibong and Chunbong. The acupressure knob is good for pressing the body's meridian points, other than the navel.

Methods for using the Belly Button Healing tool are described in Chapters 6 and 7, and the intent behind the creation of the Belly Button Healing tool is explained in Chapter 8.

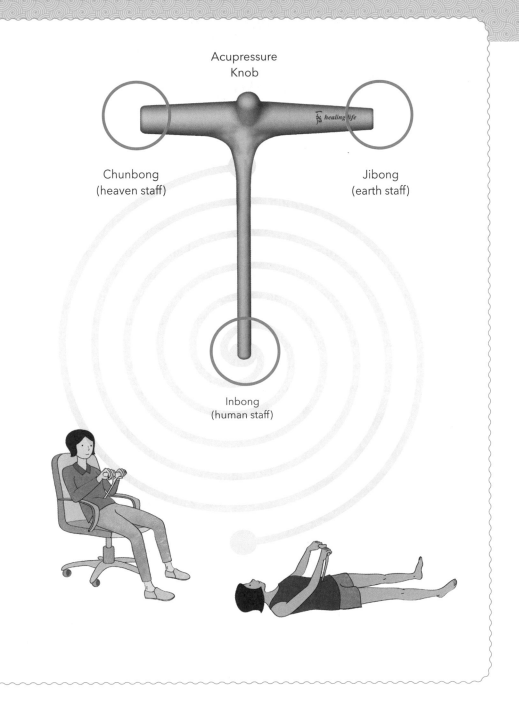

Acupressure
Knob

Chunbong
(heaven staff)

Jibong
(earth staff)

Inbong
(human staff)

CHAPTER 6

Belly Button Breathing

Self Belly Button Breathing

Belly Button Healing Step 1 is Belly Button Breathing. With Belly Button Breathing, you promote good energy and blood circulation, increase vitality, and induce relaxation of body and mind by concentrating on your exhalations as you rhythmically and mindfully press your navel with your hand or the Belly Button Healing Wand.

It is great to make a habit of Belly Button Healing because you can do it whenever you get the opportunity, especially during short breaks at work.

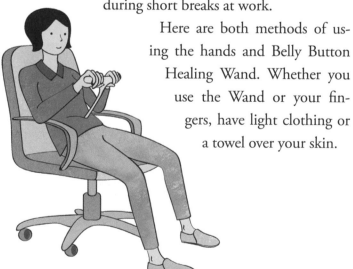

Here are both methods of using the hands and Belly Button Healing Wand. Whether you use the Wand or your fingers, have light clothing or a towel over your skin.

Using the Hands

1. Sit in a chair or lie on the floor. When sitting in a chair, lean your upper body comfortably against the back of it.

2. Gently rub your abdomen clockwise with your palm for a minute to relax your body and mind.

3. Place the three middle fingertips of both hands on your navel. Relax your shoulders and press your navel rhythmically, repeatedly, and mindfully.

4. Exhale in sharp, short breaths through your mouth or nose at this time. The relaxing effect is greater if you emphasize your outgoing breath.

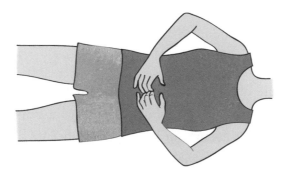

5. Do about 100 to 300 repetitions at once. This should take one to three minutes. It's better to do this frequently in short bursts than to do it once for a long time.

6. When you've finished pressing your belly button, spend at least a couple of minutes focusing on your body while you breathe comfortably as you imagine life energy entering your abdomen through your belly button. You may feel energy sensations such as tingling, heaviness leaving, cold releasing, or warmth that spreads from your abdomen to your whole body.

7. Try to feel what other changes are happening in your body, from your belly and fingertips to the tips of your toes. Then, feel your breathing deepening automatically as you become more aware and relaxed.

Using the Belly Button Healing Wand

1. Sit in a chair or lie on the floor. When sitting in a chair, lean your upper body comfortably against its back.

2. Gently rub your abdomen clockwise with your palm for a minute to relax your body and mind.

3. Place the end of the longest and thinnest part of the Belly Button Healing Wand, the Inbong, against your belly button. The tip of it fits in your belly button since it's similar in size. In that position, hold the other two ends with your

hands, and press your belly button with the Healing Life, repeatedly pulling it toward your body. Relax the tension in your shoulders, chest, and abdomen as much as possible at this time.

You'll discover that the thinnest part of the wand is bent slightly. If you use it with the curve downward, you'll feel the wand pressing vertically into your belly button, and if you use it with the curve upward, you'll get the feeling that it's pressing slightly downward from top to bottom. Both of these positions are useful and appropriate. Use whichever position you prefer and that is right for your condition.

Additionally, instead of only pressing your belly button in a vertical direction, you may apply pressure with the wand tilted 45 degrees, which allows you to do Belly Button Healing in a more varied, effective way.

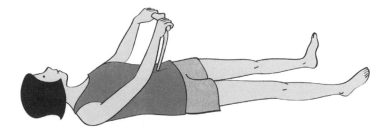

4. The rest of the process is the same as the one for using the hands described previously.

Partner Healing with Belly Button Breathing

You can use the Belly Button Breathing described before as a healing method you apply to other people. When you perform Belly Button Healing on someone who is experiencing it for the first time, use your hands instead of the Belly Button Healing Wand. When you perform Belly Button Healing on another person, you should use the tool carefully and only after fully developing a sense for it by first using it on your own body.

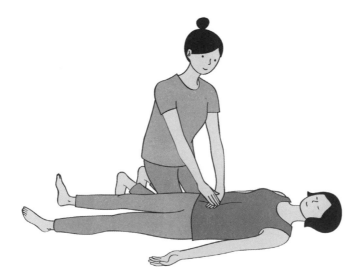

When you perform Belly Button Healing on someone who has very stiff intestines, you should release their tension first. They will feel more pain in their abdomen if you press on their navel when they're tense. If the healer gently circles a hand around the abdomen of the receiver, who is lying down, or, holding the ends of both of the receiver's feet, shakes their legs side to side, it will help relax their body and mind. Dahn-jon Tapping and Intestinal Exercise, which will be introduced later, are good to use as preparatory steps for the receiver to do before Belly Button Healing.

For Healers

1. Sit beside the person who will receive the healing.

2. Rub your palms together to activate the energy between them, then bring your palms close to the receiver's face, sending her warm healing energy.

3. With about three inches of space between your hands and the receiver's body, sweep your palms several times from head to toe through her energy field. If you do this, the receiver will feel warm energy and her energy will sink downward, helping her to relax.

4. Determine the location of the receiver's belly button by asking her to point it out with her finger.

5. Placing one hand over the other, gently press the person's navel with your fingertips.

6. Press until you feel a pulse in the person's navel with your fingertips, and press their navel repeatedly and gently unless the receiver complains of pain.

7. If the receiver complains of pain, first gently relax the navel and the area around it with the palm of your hand, and then attempt to press with your fingertips again.

8. Do about 100 to 300 repetitions at once. This should take one to three minutes. It's better to do this frequently in short bursts than to do it once for a long time.

9. When you're finished pressing the receiver's navel, have them focus on the changes in their body as, in a lying posture, they continue to breathe and feel the warmth in their abdomen that gradually spreads to their whole body.

10. Remain sitting beside the receiver. Relax your body and breathing comfortably as you imagine a shining, healing energy coming down into you and the receiver.

11. After the Belly Button Breathing, listen to what the receiver has to share about the changes they felt in their body and mind.

For Receivers

1. Lie comfortably with your back on the floor and your hands at your sides. Close your eyes, and relax your body.

2. When the hand of the healer touches your navel, imagine that your umbilical cord is connected to them, and accept the healing energy they send through it.

3. Exhale in sharp, short breaths through your mouth or nose when the healer presses your navel. The relaxing effect is greater if you exhale this way.

4. Concentrate completely on the feelings in your abdomen while receiving Belly Button Healing. When the healing is done, focus on the sensations you get throughout your body, such as warmth, tingling, pain, lightness, or heaviness leaving.

5. Breathe comfortably in that position. Feel your breath entering deep into your abdomen as your warm belly moves gently up and down.

CHAPTER 7
Belly Button Massage

Self Belly Button Massage

Belly Button Healing Step 2 is Belly Button Massage. This is a method of Belly Button Healing that uses your hands or the Belly Button Healing Wand to find pain points in and around your navel and resolve problems in associated parts of the body.

Belly Button Massage is a more profound method of healing than Belly Button Breathing, which is simply repetitively pressing the belly button. Deeply pressing pain points during Belly Button Massage allows you to get to your body's underlying energetic issues. Many people who have experienced the most profound effects of Belly Button Healing, such as reduced pain and tension and improved mobility, say that most of these effects were possible through Belly Button Massage.

Although Belly Button Breathing is effective for recharging your vitality quickly in your daily life, to experience the long-term effects of deep healing, it's very important to do Belly Button Massage on a regular basis. It's okay to do Belly Button Massage with your thumbs, but, if you use the Belly Button Healing Wand, you can stimulate your belly button much more easily and effectively.

Using the Hands

1. Lie down and gently rub your lower abdomen clockwise with the palm of your hand several times while relaxing your body and mind.

2. Imagine that your belly button is divided into eight sections, like a pie chart, centered on the middle of the navel. Using your thumb, go in a clockwise direction around the eight points, gently pressing down and toward each, one by one, to identify painful areas. The positions of pain points may be different each time you do Belly Button Massage.

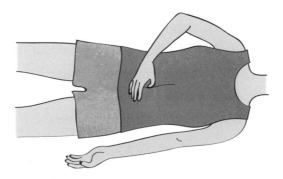

3. Gently and rapidly press the pain points you find about 10 times. If all of the pain is not released, you can repeat this two or three more times.

4. Breathe comfortably and focus on how your body feels.

Using the Belly Button Healing Wand

1. Lie down and gently rub your lower abdomen clockwise with the palm of your hand several times while relaxing your body and mind.

2. Place the end of the longest and thinnest part of the Belly Button Healing Wand against your belly button. If you want more gentle healing, you can use thicker ends of it.

   It's important that you find for yourself how deeply to press at this time. Pressing too weakly has little effect, while pressing too forcefully could have adverse effects. There will be times when you feel some pain, but it should not be excruciating or lingering. Most people can recognize the feeling of "good pain," like when you are stretching deeply or doing strength training. You should press deeply enough to feel a subtle level of pain, a sign that blockages are breaking up and releasing.

   The ideal depth will vary from person to person. If you feel pain even when you're not pressing too hard, it could mean that your abdomen is tense or that your body is in poor shape. If you feel only pressure and no pain even though you press deeply, it means your intestines and body are relatively healthy. Additionally, someone without a lot of belly fat won't have to press deeply, but someone with a lot of belly fat will need to press deeper to find the points were pain is felt.

3. Once you've developed a sense for how hard to press, you will need to find your belly button's pain points. Use the wand to press your belly button once in each of the four directions—north, south, east, and west. You may feel sharper pain while pressing in one direction than in another.

   After checking the four directions, try pressing in the eight directions, adding northwest, southwest, and so on. If you go deeper, you could even try pressing in the 12 directions. That's complicated, though, so it's enough to just check the eight directions. If you release all the pain you find, even if it's just through the eight directions, your energy and blood circulation will improve.

   Belly button pain develops because of poor energy and blood circulation. The pain you feel when you press the top of your belly button is associated with parts of your body that are above your navel. Examples are chest and throat pain, headache, and stomach illness. Pain to the

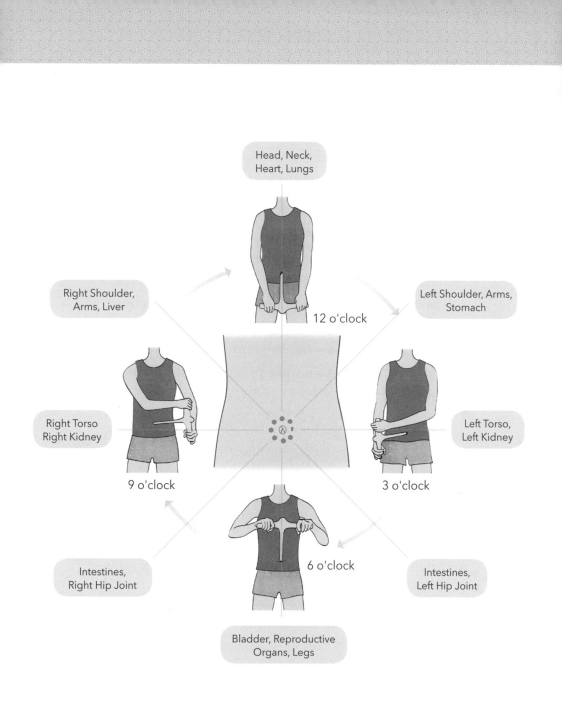

Head, Neck,
Heart, Lungs

Right Shoulder,
Arms, Liver

Left Shoulder, Arms,
Stomach

12 o'clock

Right Torso
Right Kidney

Left Torso,
Left Kidney

9 o'clock

3 o'clock

Intestines,
Right Hip Joint

Intestines,
Left Hip Joint

6 o'clock

Bladder, Reproductive
Organs, Legs

left of the belly button is associated with the stomach, the left side of the intestines, and kidneys, and pain to the right of the belly button is associated with the liver, gallbladder, right side of the intestines, and kidneys. Next, pain to the bottom of the belly button is associated with the urinary and reproductive systems, which includes the uterus and bladder. Pain felt in the eight directions is associated with pain in the left shoulder, right shoulder, left hip, and right hip.

Your priority is finding where you hurt the most. You first have to take care of the side with the most pain. For example, if you feel intense pain on the right side of your belly button, then energy and blood circulation has stagnated in associated areas on the right side of your body, which affects energy and blood circulation throughout your body.

4. Once you find pain points, focus your healing there. Place the wand on the pain point and gently press, with the wand tilted about 45 degrees in the opposite direction. Press until you feel pain to some degree using the sense acquired as described above. Repeat this exercise several times, pressing with the wand and then taking it away, and you will sense that the severity of the pain you felt at first has decreased significantly.

5. After finishing Belly Button Massage, breathe comfortably and concentrate on how the feelings in your body are changing. As your energy and blood circulation improve, you'll feel a pleasant heat spreading out through your body.

6. What's amazing about Belly Button Healing is that pain subsides as soon as you do it. Pain does not totally disappear with one application of Belly Button Healing, though. That's why you have to regularly and repeatedly perform Belly Button Healing until the knotted areas all relax, your energy and blood circulation is smooth, and your condition is restored.

Partner Healing with Belly Button Massage

You can use Belly Button Massage with other people as well. A good subject for Belly Button Healing is someone who says that they feel a lot of pain after their belly button is pressed. Performing Belly Button Healing on such a person can have a great effect. When you perform Belly Button Healing on someone who is experiencing it for the first time, use your hands instead of the Belly Button Healing Wand.

For Healers

1. Gently rub the receiver's lower abdomen clockwise with the palm of your hand for about one minute to relax the receiver's body and mind.

2. Determine the receiver's physical condition by asking them to tell you where in their body they normally experience discomfort or health problems.

3. Rub your palms together to activate the energy between them, then bring your palms close to the receiver's face, sending it warm healing energy.

4. With about three inches of space between your hands and the receiver's body, sweep your palms several times from head to toe through the receiver's energy field. If you do this, the receiver will feel warm energy and her energy will sink downward, helping her relax.

5. Determine the location of the receiver's belly button by asking her to point it out with her finger.

6. As you gently press the receiver's navel, check whether or not she is tense. Pain means that she is tense.

7. Imagine that the receiver's belly button is divided into eight sections like a pie chart centered on the middle of the navel. Using your thumb, go in a clockwise direction around the eight points, gently pressing down and

toward each, one by one, to identify painful areas. Have the receiver tell you where any pain is as you press down. You can identify the points by associating them with the numbers around a clock dial.

8. When you find a pain point, press it gently with your thumb, maintaining the pressure for 10 seconds before taking your thumb away. Repeat this several times. Then massage the area of the pain point, relaxing it.

9. The pain is not always completely released in a single session, so verify the extent of the pain every time you do Belly Button Massage. The positions of pain points may also be different each time.

10. When the receiver feels comfortable about using the Belly Button Healing Wand, you can let the receiver press their belly button with the wand.

11. When you're finished with Belly Button Massage, have the receiver focus on the changes in their body as, in a lying posture, they continue to breathe. They may feel warmth in their abdomen that spreads through their body, or sensations such as tingling, lightness, or heaviness leaving. These sensations are evidence of energy releasing.

12. At this time, the healer also sits beside the receiver, controlling their breathing and imagining a shining, healing energy coming down into themselves and the receiver.

13. After the Belly Button Massage, listen to what the receiver has to share about the changes they felt in their body and mind.

For Receivers

1. Lie comfortably with your back on the floor.

2. Close your eyes and relax your body.

3. When the hand of the person doing the healing touches your navel, imagine that an umbilical cord is connected to them, and accept the healing energy that they send through it.

4. Using the numbers on the face of an imaginary clock over your navel as a reference, tell the healer the locations where you feel pain when your belly button is pressed. If you feel pain or other responses in other parts of your body, tell the healer about it immediately.

5. When the healer massages a pain point, stay as relaxed as you can as you focus on your outgoing breath.

6. When the Belly Button Massage is done, breathe comfortably, observing the changes in your body and mind. Feel energy sensations such as warmth, tingling, or heaviness traveling through or out of your body.

CHAPTER 8
Healing Life, Healing the Earth

After discovering the powerful healing potential of the belly button for myself, I wanted to share it with as many people as possible through Belly Button Healing. I knew that they would have to experience it directly for themselves because it can't be understood through words alone. I thought hard about whether there might be some way for everyone to experience the effects of Belly Button Healing easily, which lead me to create the Belly Button Healing Wand.

I was researching Hwangchil, an herb also known as *Dendropanax morbifera*, which has a variety of healing effects, when I discovered a Hwangchil tree branch shaped perfectly for belly button stimulation. It was shaped like a T, and could be easily grasped by both hands as the bottom part was used to push into the belly button. Up until that time, I had only pressed my belly button with my hand as I did Belly Button Healing. My arms hurt, and not enough force went into it. But when I took a branch of the Hwangchil tree and used it to press my belly button, I discovered that the effects were incredible. So we produced the Belly Button Healing tool we have now based on the shape of that tree limb.

I named the tool "Healing Life" because I wanted this wand to be a tool for more than just healing the body. Rather,

I envisioned a tool that could be used to heal people's lives, and, if used to its full potential, to heal the earth.

The earth, which is suffering from all kinds of environmental degradation, urgently needs healing, now more than ever before. If the planet is to be healed, though, people must first heal themselves, since we are ultimately the cause of the earth's contamination. Humanity is sick—physically, mentally, and spiritually—and that has made the earth sick. I believe that true planetary healing will only begin when people recover their original state of health, happiness, and peace. From there, it can spread to all the earth from person to person. Healthy people can share health; happy people can share positive energy; peaceful people will bring peace to those around them.

How, then, can people be healed? They need methods for restoring and managing their mental as well as physical health, and they need methods for awakening their life energy and for living according to the central values of life. All of these are contained in Belly Button Healing.

The Key to Life Is Emotional Control

To heal our lives, we must make management of our emotions a priority. We are living in countless waves of emotions every day. Our emotions are produced by our bodies and minds, and they directly affect the condition of our bodies and minds.

The part of our bodies that exhibit the quickest reaction, especially when we are under stress, is our intestines. Oriental medicine practitioners also believe that specific emotions are linked to specific organs. For example, venting too much anger damages your liver; over-excitement damages your heart; thinking and worrying too much damages your stomach; being too sorrowful damages your lungs; and being too fearful damages your kidneys. Conversely, the state of health of the organs also influences emotion. If your liver is weak, you will be irritable and show a lot of anger. Those with weak hearts often can't relax their minds and talk too much. Those with weak stomachs are afflicted by worrying and racing thoughts. Those with weak lungs are often depressed and sorrowful, even over trivial situations, while those with weak kidneys are fearful and startled even by small noises.

When you're caught in such an emotional state, your feelings create a plethora of thoughts and judgments, and the energy of your emotions grows stronger and heavier. If emotional energy continues to accumulate without being released, ultimately problems develop in the energy and blood circulation of the intestines, leading to various psychogenic diseases.

The problem is that people don't know effective ways to

control their emotions. For example, when people experience a surge of anger, they generally have two ways of dealing with it—either they will express the anger outwardly or they will suppress it. Stifling those feelings keeps the energy of anger bottled up inside your body, and, as a result, the energy has a negative effect on you physically. However, outwardly expressing yourself whenever you're angry is also bad for your personal relationships. Moreover, such behavior stimulates the emotions of others, which could cause even greater problems.

What, then, should you do at such times? You should consider ways to understand your emotions as energy and to process that energy constructively. You can begin by perceiving the energy in your body not as thought, but as sensation. If you focus on your chest when you're angry or sad, you'll clearly perceive a feeling of heaviness and blockage there. That is the sensation of heavy, stagnated emotional energy. You have to discharge the energy from your body to keep from bottling it up inside.

Belly Button Healing is the best method for discharging and purifying energy that has stagnated in your organs. As you repeatedly pump your belly button, you can send the accumulated emotional energy out of your body with your exhaled breath. What's more, if you gently press the pain points of your belly button, you will be able to feel the release of stagnant emotions from deep inside your body, along with your physical pain.

When we are mired in emotion, our ability to read other's emotions or to accurately observe situations drops precipitously. So our mind becomes narrow and the ability to be tolerant declines. Clashes between our emotions and those of others make it difficult to have good personal relationships. This, in turn, leads to familial and societal conflict. Failure to manage our emotions is one of main causes of unhappiness and discontent in the world.

Living their lives with a belly full of unpurified feelings, modern people end up collecting too many emotional scars. Since their insides are filled with emotions that haven't healed, they are afraid to meet other people. They build walls and hide from others to protect their own emotions from being disturbed. Ours has become a world where people are afraid of people.

For this reason, we should vigilantly guard against being mired in negative emotions. Words spoken when we are stuck in such emotions become toxic and murderous weapons. Just think of all the negative information and expressions flowing through our society right now through media and the Internet! Such negative information scars people's hearts and makes their brains whither, which in turn puts even more distance between them and their true nature. Every day, it seems to get worse and worse. We all must rediscover our true selves if we hope to reverse this trend.

I developed the Belly Button Healing method and wand

to make the world a place where all people recover their true nature and integrity, allowing them to open their hearts to each other without fear, to communicate, and to love each other. The Healing Life is a tool designed to enable us to heal ourselves inside and to become individuals filled with happiness and peace that emanate from our inner being.

Every evening before you go to sleep, press your belly button with the Healing Life wand. The waves of emotion that come with the events of the day will subside, and your brain will become clearer. Then, as you look back on the things you experienced during the day, unresolved feelings will find their solutions, and your body and mind will become relaxed. Also, your brain will excrete the hormone serotonin, which will brighten your mood. You'll be able to discover your true, unfeigned nature in that process.

How to Attain a Meditative State Naturally

For everyone, the past is something that is gone; it is beyond return. And even one minute from now is merely the future, which has not yet arrived. No one knows what will happen in even one minute. We exist only now, in the present. Yet, whether consciously or unconsciously, most of us suffer from what has happened in the irreversible past, and we worry about what will happen in the future. If your brain is continuously enslaved by anxieties and worries about the past or future, you must emancipate it immediately.

Techniques for managing the brain are crucial in these times when we're flooded with countless forms of information. We have been taught how to use computers, but no one teaches us how to manage and use our brains. Thought and knowledge are not enough to manage the brain well. You must be able to feel the state of your own brain, and you must acquire a sense that allows you to return to your brain's original, pure state, a state beyond the influence of emotions or information. This state of consciousness is referred to as the "zero-point state."

Managing the brain is like managing our weight. When you step on your bathroom scale, you will not get an accurate reading if the scale is set to five instead of zero. Likewise, we can judge all circumstances accurately from a zero-point brain state. If the needle on your brain-state scale has moved away from zero, it means you're mired in negative or positive emotions. In a zero-point state, consciousness is free of attachment because it is neutral. Because of that, you feel free. So, if you really want to become free and peaceful, you have no choice but to recover your zero point. Then, you can sincerely and authentically commune with yourself and others.

Of course, as we live our lives, we might become caught up in emotions and influenced by skewed information at any time. The question is whether we will continue in that state, subjecting ourselves to stress, or quickly emerge from it. We need technology that allows us to come out of that condition and return to our zero point when we want to. This kind of technology would allow us to manage our information and emotions, and, furthermore, to manage our lives.

One such method is meditation. Just meditating aimlessly, however, does not allow immediate recovery of the zero-point state. Often, when we sit down to meditate, all kinds of thoughts come to mind, one after another. If you sit for 30 minutes in such a state, although it looks like you're meditating on the outside, it's not actually meditation. For those without years of careful training, that situation is common.

For creating a meditative state, a zeroed state, Belly Button Healing is one of the easiest and most convenient tools that I know. When you're pressing your belly button, you naturally focus on the feelings in your body. Your consciousness, which was once directed entirely outward, comes back into your body. And your energy, which had been driven above your head by all your thoughts and worries, sinks into your lower abdomen, the center of your body. You escape from your useless worries and thoughts, naturally achieving a meditative state, a zeroed state, without intentionally trying. As mentioned previously, the effects of Belly Button Healing are so amazing that it is no exaggeration to say that five minutes of this practice is equal to 30 minutes of deep breathing.

The super-simple secret to attaining a meditative state is found in the belly button, and in Healing Life. No matter how well you understand these principles, they are useless unless you actually make them a part of your daily life. Healing Life is convenient because, if you grab and apply it, you can immediately experience the effects of Belly Button Healing. This is why I believe that Healing Life is like a master key allowing us to open the door of healing in our bodies, minds, and lives, a door through which we can progress toward healing the earth, as well.

From Belly Button Healing to Earth Management

A world where humans and nature are truly respected, a world of healing where love for humanity and love for the earth are realized—this is the concept called "Earth Management" that I dream of. I have put that dream into Healing Life.

I believe that the era of the global village, a time of a peaceful, mature civilization, will come when the consciousness of humankind awakens. The defining characteristic of that consciousness is a spirit that has returned to zero point.

Only after we have recovered a zeroed state free of attachments will communication, true communion, and lasting unity finally be possible between individuals, between religions, and between nations. Then we can go forward together toward a common vision of Earth Management, the greatest dream of humankind.

But, if we realistically hope to achieve that, everyone must learn the sense and techniques that allow them to return to a zeroed state at any time. Only then will we know unequivocally the importance and value of our True Selves and preciousness of our individual lives. Only then will we be able to accurately check whether our intended direction is the right one. With the hope that all people will learn this, I have been developing and teaching various mind-body training methods, including Brain Education, for about 40 years. Hoping to increase the speed at which these things are realized, I was led to develop Healing Life.

Healing Life looks like a simple product, but it has a story, and it has a spirit. It contains all the principles of Korean traditional mind-body training, which are at the core of the Brain Education that I've been teaching. It contains the spirit and resolve to save myself, other people, and humanity, a spirit that I've kept in my heart from the time I first taught a stroke patient in a park about 40 years ago.

Moreover, if you are willing to experience the practice deeply, you'll be able to feel that you're connected to the history of human origins and to fundamental life energy through the belly button. I'm in the habit of saying that to know the value of the belly button is to know your own value, the value of life, and, furthermore, the value of the earth.

What is the reason we've come into this world? And what is the reason we've come to the earth now, in the twenty-first century? I believe that the answers depend on the choices of each person. The value of your life isn't set; you choose and create it for yourself.

I recommend that you open your heart and try making this the philosophy of your life: "I have chosen the earth, and the earth has chosen me. My birth wasn't random; I have come here through the great providence of nature. I came to this planet because earth of the twenty-first century earnestly needed me, and I exist on this planet because I can do something for the earth and for nature." After you've deliberately chosen your life's values in this way, you'll feel the sacredness of your life, and the undeniable significance in your life, which until now you may have wasted, wandering in search of a worthy goal.

Your mind is the one that chooses this. That mind may occasionally be narrower than the eye of a needle, but it can also grow large enough to contain the earth and the universe, depending on your choice. We humans have such mysterious minds. But people's minds have dwindled. They have been diminished by the state, they have been diminished by religion, they have been diminished by erroneous education and information, and they have been diminished by personal relationships. The creator has given humanity the power to choose and create value. That is what distinguishes humans from other animals, and that is why humans have a special role to play in the development of life in the cosmos.

I hope you, like many before you, will be able to discover the power of your mind, and to choose and create your life's true values. Let's choose lives of healing ourselves, other people, and the earth, and let's begin by encountering our lives authentically as we press our belly buttons. Any great awakening and action in this world ultimately begins inside us.

"From the belly button to the earth, from Belly Button Healing to Earth Management." These are not two things, but one, and they are not separate, but inevitable, natural, and reasonable steps. When we are healed and our lives are healed, we can also heal our sick planet. Let's begin that healing in our belly buttons.

The time of the belly button has now come. I sincerely hope, as belly-button culture becomes known in the world, that countless people will awaken to know that humanity's hope lies in moving "from the belly button to the earth," and that everyone will join together to create a common vision of love for humanity and love for the earth.

CHAPTER 9

Healthy Belly Exercises

Belly Button Healing is not the only way to stimulate your abdomen to improve digestion, circulation, immunity, and body alignment. Other exercises, which I have been teaching since before I discovered the benefits of navel stimulation, also have these holistic effects. All of them involve deeper and broader movement of the abdomen than Belly Button Healing.

Like Belly Button Healing, these exercises release energy blockages in your abdomen, pelvis, and chest so that your energy can circulate healthfully. With healthy energy circulation, your head stays clear and cool, improving your brain function, and the organs keep warm, helping them work at their best. They encourage blood, food, and lymph to move through your abdomen so that toxins are better eliminated and enough nutrients and oxygen get to all parts of your body.

You can use these exercises on their own or before performing Belly Button Healing to loosen and relax the abdomen. Combine them all together or pick and choose the ones that work best for your body and schedule. If you would like to combine all of them, the best order in which to do them is Dahnjon Tapping to warm your abdomen and draw your focus there, Intestinal Exercise to loosen the organs and fascia in your abdomen and remove energy blockages, and then Intestinal Massage to find and remove deeper tension and blockages.

Dahnjon Tapping

Dahnjon Tapping, which involves using the palms of the hands to tap the abdomen below the navel, is an exercise that effectively activates intestinal function by directly stimulating and vibrating the intestines.

Strengthening the Dahnjon has an effect similar to starting up an energy generator in the body. When the energy of the Dahnjon is activated, the abdomen, hands, and feet are always warm, digestion is good, and the body's different circulatory functions operate smoothly. You naturally sit up straighter and think more clearly.

You can prevent your intestines from being stiff if you develop a habit of doing Dahnjon Tapping whenever you have time during the day. Also, doing Dahnjon Tapping for about one to two minutes before doing Belly Button Healing increases heat in the abdomen and releases tension in the body, which increases the effectiveness of Belly Button Healing.

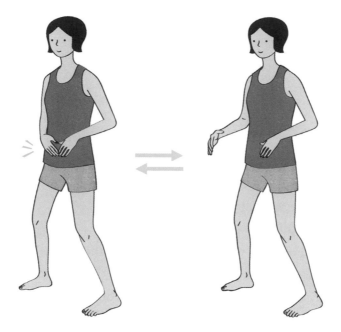

1. Stand with your feet shoulder-width apart.

2. Place your palms lightly on your lower abdomen and bend your knees slightly. When you bend your knees slightly, your Dahnjon will tense as your body's center of gravity forms there.

3. Tap below your navel with the palms of your hands. It's easy for your shoulders and arms to become tense with this position. Tap using the bounce of your arms to keep your shoulders as relaxed as possible.

4. When you feel heat in your Dahnjon, continue by tapping your upper abdomen and sides, too.

5. Bending your upper body forward slightly, also tap your lower back.

6. Do Dahnjon Tapping as often as you can based on your schedule. One recommendation is to start out with 300 repetitions, either at one time or spread throughout your day.

7. Another version of Dahnjon Tapping is to use the palm side of your loose fists. For stronger and more concentrated stimulation, use the pinky side of your fists. Try these variations and see which one has the greatest effect on you.

Intestinal Exercise

Intestinal Exercise involves repeatedly pulling and pushing your lower belly in and out, releasing tension throughout your abdomen and promoting intestinal health.

About 30 to 40 percent of the blood in your whole body flows in your abdomen, which is why doing Intestinal Exercise has the effect of increasing your blood circulation. Additionally, Intestinal Exercise will increase your body temperature enough to make you sweat, even though you're only moving your belly.

While the pumping motion is similar to doing Belly Button Breathing without your hands or a Healing Wand, the movement accesses more of the lower abdomen, around your Dahnjon. With many repetitions, it also increases your core muscle strength, helping to keep your body aligned.

Intestinal Exercise is an excellent exercise you can actively recommend to people who are always short of energy because of chronic hypothermia, whose intestinal function is weak, who have given up making a habit of exercise, or who say they can't find time to exercise. The simple movement of pulling and pushing your lower abdominal wall can be done in any posture at any time, even as you are performing other tasks such as working at a computer, watching TV, or driving a car. It is especially useful for circulating your blood and energy when you need to sit for long periods of time.

If you do Intestinal Exercise in specific postures, then it

will have a greater effect. The following 10 basic forms change your body posture in a variety of ways to alter the effect of the exercise. You can do each posture on its own, or combine all 10 in a sequence for maximum benefit.

Guidelines for Intestinal Exercises

- Set a goal of doing a certain number of repetitions during the day, and then do some whenever you get the chance.

- Although Intestinal Exercise is a very simple movement of pushing out and pulling in the abdomen, the most important of these two is the pulling in motion. When pulling in, pull as if the front wall of your abdomen is trying to touch your back. If you pull in strongly, the pushing out motion will happen naturally.

- The effects may vary somewhat depending on the speed with which you do Intestinal Exercise. Doing Intestinal Exercise quickly greatly stimulates your intestinal peristalsis, improving your energy and blood circulation. If you do Intestinal Exercise slowly and deeply, it has the same effects as deep abdominal breathing, so energy accumulates in your Dahnjon and your whole body grows warmer.

- Be sure to keep your arms and shoulders relaxed when you do Intestinal Exercise, just as when you do Dahnjon Tapping. When you pull your abdomen inward, check in a mirror to see whether your shoulders are rising without your realizing it. If you do, consciously relax them. However, if it's difficult to keep your shoulders relaxed even when you are aware of your tension, it's okay to do the exercise with your arms hanging at your sides, without placing your hands on your belly.

- The first time you do Intestinal Exercise or when you have built-up tension in your body, you may experience pain when you pull in your abdomen. If this happens, gently massage the place that hurts and wait for the pain to subside. When the pain is gone, gently resume.

Intestinal Exercise Form 1

1. Stand with your feet shoulder-width apart and arch your lower back and bend your knees slightly.

2. Place your palms gently on your lower abdomen with the tips of your thumbs meeting over your navel and the sides of the tips of your pointer fingers meeting below that, forming a flat triangle with your hands.

3. Using your abdominal muscles, pull the area of your abdomen below your navel in toward your back as far as possible. Exhale as you pull inward.

4. Then, relaxing as much as possible, push it out slightly. Inhale when you push outward.

5. Repeat this pulling and pushing motion fluidly.

6. When you pull your belly inward, it's even better if you also repeatedly contract your anal sphincter.

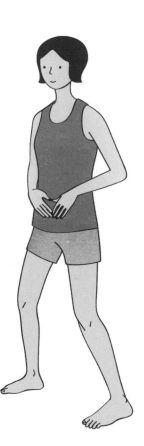

Intestinal Exercise Form 2

Standing as in Form 1, straighten your knees and bend forward, placing your palms on the floor. Move your abdomen fluidly in and out in this posture. It's okay if your hands don't completely touch the floor. Just bend forward as far as you can. Don't do this posture if you have pain in your lower back.

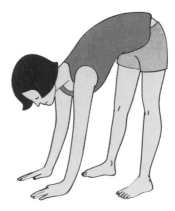

Intestinal Exercise Form 3

From the posture of Form 2, kneel on the ground, placing your palms on the floor and supporting your upper body with your arms. Your hips and shoulders should make 90-degree angles with your back. Raise your head and upper body so that your lumbar vertebrae form a natural curve. Do Intestinal Exercise in this position.

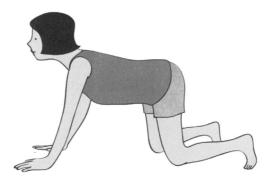

Intestinal Exercise Form 4

From the posture of Form 3, raise your upper body and do Intestinal Exercise with only your knees touching the floor. Gently place your palms on your lower abdomen in the same triangle position as in Form 1 and follow the same instructions for Intestinal Exercise. Kneel on a yoga mat or a cushion if the floor is too hard.

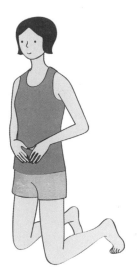

Intestinal Exercise Form 5

From the posture of Form 4, relax and sit on the floor with your legs crossed or in a half-lotus position. Do Intestinal Exercise with your palms in a triangle on your lower abdomen.

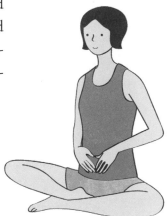

Intestinal Exercise Form 6

From the posture of Form 5, lie down with your knees bent and the soles of your feet and your back touching the floor. Put your knees together and spread your feet shoulder-width apart. Gently place your hands on your lower abdomen, and do Intestinal Exercise.

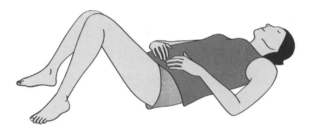

Intestinal Exercise Form 7

From the posture of Form 6, turn to lie on your left side. Support your head with your upper left arm and place your right hand on your lower abdomen. Bend your knees so that your body is slightly curled up, and do Intestinal Exercise in this position.

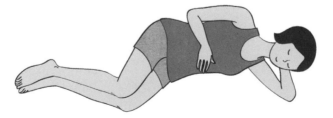

Intestinal Exercise Form 8

From the posture of Form 7, turn to lie on your right side. Support your head with your upper right arm and place your left hand on your lower abdomen. Bend your knees so that your body is slightly curled up, and do Intestinal Exercise in this position.

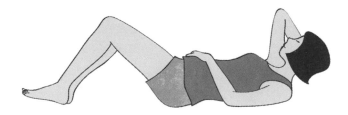

Intestinal Exercise Form 9

From the posture of Form 8, turn so that you are again lying with your back and feet touching the floor and your knees in the air. Pushing up on the soles of your feet, raise your hips until you make a straight line from your knees to your shoulder blades. Gently place your palms on your lower abdomen, and do Intestinal Exercise.

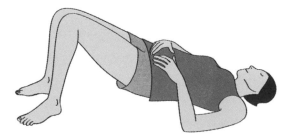

Intestinal Exercise Form 10

Slowly stand up and adopt the posture of Form 1. From here, bend your upper body forward about 30 degrees, and do Intestinal Exercise.

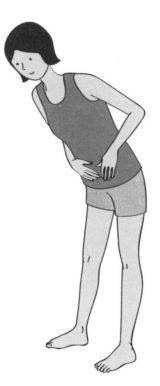

Intestinal Massage

Intestinal Massage is a healing method that improves intestinal function and increases vitality in the whole body by using the hands to massage and relax stiffness throughout the abdomen. If you do Intestinal Massage along with Belly Button Healing, you can get a greater effect by combining the light, concentrated focus of Belly Button Healing with the deeper, more widely spread pressing of Intestinal Massage.

With its shallow movements, Belly Button Healing may impart its benefits by stimulating nerves around the belly button, while Intestinal Massage has a deeper, mechanical effect on peristalsis and circulation.

With both Belly Button Healing and Intestinal Massage, the Belly Button Healing Wand can be used to mimic the actions of hands. Implementing this tool makes both methods easier and more effective.

Your intention and attitude also affect the effectiveness of any form of healing. Even if you haven't been able to accumulate that much experience or skill, massaging with caring intention will help guide your movements. If you focus on the person receiving healing and move your hands with presence of mind and a caring attitude, you will also convey warm energy to them. That alone will enable the receiver to experience comfort and peace of body and mind.

Quietly placing one hand on the receiver's navel can be enough to cause burping or rumbling in their intestines as they relax. Healing begins the instant you open your heart and share energy. There are several ways to do Intestinal Massage.

- Massage with fingers: Massage the abdomen using the pads of the fingers, not allowing the fingernails to touch the receiver.

- Massage with palms: Gently press and massage the abdomen using the palms of the hands.

- Massage with palms of overlapped hands: Use both palms to press and massage more deeply.

- Press with palms and shake: Gently shake the abdomen and hips from side to side when intestines are tense.

- Massage with fingers and the whole palms: Hold the abdomen with your fingers and palms and release.

Use the methods above as appropriate for the condition of the intestines of the person receiving the massage.

You can start with rubbing and then shaking the abdomen for overall relaxation. Then, as with Belly Button Massage, gently press with your fingertips in a clockwise direction around the whole abdomen to find the most painful and/or stiff areas. Ask the receiver to describe how they feel as you press down. Finally, focus on areas that are especially stiff. Use

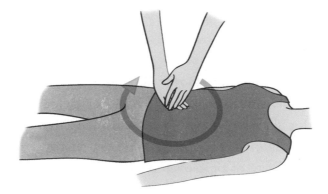

the various hand techniques above to work out any tension. Choose the appropriate techniques based on the condition of the receiver's abdomen. Use gentler motions if they have pain, and press more deeply in cases where they have more, but not painful, tension.

3 Dietary Tips for Intestinal Health

1. Ingest probiotics.

Probiotics became widely known when Russian biologist Ilya Ilyich Mechnikov discovered that the reason Bulgarians are long-lived is that they consume fermented milk containing large quantities of lactobacilli. It's important to consume an adequate quantity of probiotics because they increase the number of beneficial bacteria and suppress harmful bacteria in the gut. The best approach is to eat fermented foods daily, like yogurt, kefir, kimchi, sauerkraut, and kombucha, along with probiotic supplements.

2. Increase your consumption of dietary fiber.

It's important to consume dietary fiber, which is food for probiotic bacteria and helps to keep the gut free of debris. Dietary fiber is a polymer substance that is difficult for digestive enzymes to break down. It is found in the cell walls of plants and is also in the husks of plant seeds. Large amounts are contained in grains, beans, nuts, and mushrooms, as well as in fruits and vegetables. Too much fiber, however, can cause bloating and/or diahrea, so adjust your fiber intake according to your own body's needs.

3. Limit sugar intake.

Continuous, excessive consumption of sugar leads to chronic diseases like obesity, hypertension, and diabetes, and also impedes brain function. Too much sugar gives rise to inflammatory substances that suppress the immune system and obstruct balance in the enteric ecosystem. Not only should you cut down on the actual sugar you put in food, but you should also reduce your consumption of soft drinks, fruit juices with added sugar, and refined carbohydrates like those found in flour.

CHAPTER 10
Stories of Healing

Belly Button Healing is notable among the hundreds of natural healing techniques that I have developed because of its profound simplicity and surprising level of effectiveness. Thousands of people worldwide have benefited from Belly Button Healing, and many inspiring stories have emerged.

Even if you don't have any specific health issues, you are likely to be amazed at the relaxation and the increased energy that you feel through Belly Button Healing. We have heard about recovery from an incredible array of ailments: lower back pain, headache, cold hands and feet, chronic fatigue, just to name a few. Of course, Belly Button Healing is not meant to replace medical care, but it is clear that it can greatly assist the body in the process of recovery. In the next few pages, you will meet some of the people making physical and mental changes in their lives with the help of Belly Button Healing.

Pain Gone in My Lower Back

I had a very novel experience with Belly Button Healing. I took part in an event at a time when my lower back was killing me, so I took about five minutes and did Belly Button Healing. Afterward, my back didn't hurt, even though I sat for over two hours in a chair at the event. My lower back felt so good that I didn't need a cane when I got up from my seat after the event was over. Before, I didn't realize that the effect of stimulating the navel could be so great. I recommend to everyone that they make Belly Button Healing a part of their everyday life. I think this could be a very simple, effective method of managing your health, one that allows you to protect your health and the health of your family.

— *Suseong Lee, former Prime Minister, South Korea*

Recurring Headache Went Away

Beginning two or three years ago, I've had headaches, almost without fail, whenever I've had my period. Generally, the left side of my head would throb for about two days, and then, just about when I thought it had calmed down, the pain would sneak over and start pounding the right side of my head. During the four or five days I would suffer from a headache like this, simply maintaining my daily life, eating and sleeping, even working, were extremely difficult.

Without missing a beat, the headaches came during my recent period, too. It was a time when I had to do some important work, so I was more worried about my schedule than about the suffering the headaches cause. That was the day when I went to get Belly Button Healing. I got the healing lying down, and, before going to bed that evening, I did Belly Button Healing for about 10 minutes by myself, and then fell asleep. The headaches continued the next day, but the pain was much lighter than at other times. I did Belly Button Healing whenever I got the chance during the day, and I carefully did Intestinal Massage in bed, too, before going to sleep.

Getting up the next morning, I realized something when I was getting ready for work. The headaches had totally disappeared. That was a first for me. When they'd come, they'd usually last at least three days. Now, though, the headaches had left with their tails between their legs. I was so thrilled I wanted to laugh.

Now, when I get ready for bed, the first thing I do is Belly Button Healing. When I get ready for work in the mornings, I never forget to put my Belly Button Healing Wand in my bag. When my eyes get tired and I feel a little worn out working at the office, I do Belly Button Healing, leaning back in my chair with my eyes closed. When I do this for two or three minutes and then straighten my lower back and do abdominal breathing, I feel my condition improving right away.

— Yeogyeong Kim, South Korea

Energy Movement Deepened Breath and Released Pain

With 100 two-thumb navel pushes, I felt a sharp line of pain in my liver area and a squishing sound in my abdomen. When I stopped, the liver pain went through my right front-side throat, and my right back jaw and teeth felt pressure. As I write, the sharp pressure feeling is poking here and there throughout my lower body. My legs and feet have a buzzing feeling and feel more open and warm. Also, pressing my belly button naturally let me exhale during the process. The feeling of the movement became very clear, crisp, and fast—like the perfect Intestinal Exercise. My breathing naturally deepened during the practice, and afterward, my abdomen felt alive and refreshed as it continued the breath cycle automatically.

– Sandra Scheer, Miami, FL

Heart Burn Relieved

Today I worked with someone who came to me with very bad heart burn from eating spicy food for lunch. Her stomach was very tight, and her chest was in deep pain. After sending her calming energy into her stomach, I gently but firmly pressed the eight points in her belly button, rested, then repeated the eight points a total of four times. Her stomach growled a lot, and her abdominal temperature regulated. Within about five minutes, she was completely fine again; it was really amazing!

– Christie Jensen, Kirkland, WA

Shoulder Pain Released

I have a frozen right shoulder, which has been bothering me because of the limitation in the movement of my shoulder. Recently, I had an opportunity to receive Belly Button Healing from Ilchi Lee. I had no pain in my left shoulder while I was waiting in line for his healing. However, as soon as my shoulder touched the massage table, the sudden sharp pain caused me shortness of breath. The pain went away after the first round of Belly Button Healing. I felt my upper left chest was lighter. Then, when Ilchi Lee touched my shoulder, I felt a lot of pain on my collarbone, which I never had before. Now, my chest is lighter.

I had my appendix removed in 2014. I felt a moderate tension on the lower right edge of my belly button during the healing. Two hours later, I felt like a swirling energy released inside of my lower right. Another two hours later, that area started to awaken; I felt a little stingy pain. I felt the energy from the healing still circulating inside of my body, especially around my waist.

After Ilchi Lee's healing on my shoulder, an hour later, I felt the soreness release down to my upper arm, and after some time, it went down to my ring finger. I felt the same sensation throughout today. I am very excited about all these healing effects that I'm experiencing with Belly Button Healing.

– Ba Ha, Rockville, MD

Improved Mobility Without Discomfort

I have not been able to use my body for a while the way I used to, since hurting two discs in my lower back. It improved after 10 sessions of acupuncture, but I still felt stiffness and pressure squashing down vertebrae in that area. I was skeptical about a short time of Belly Button Healing making a difference, but immediately after, circulation in my lower body improved, my hips relaxed, and lower spine elongated, creating space between vertebrae, therefore improving my mobility without discomfort.

One more thing: my right leg, which was shorter since I was seven years old after I broke my thigh, got longer. And my tailbone was twisted to one side, and it's better now. When I sit, both sitting bones feel even, and both legs feel more even. My digestive system is better, and I have less constipation. I am maintaining my energy much better.

— *Magdalena Szara, Mount Prospect, IL*

No More Coffee Cravings

My intent when I first started Belly Button Healing was to heal my right hip. It is healing; I have more movement and less pain. The unexpected changes are no must-have-coffee craving when I wake up, improvement in focus, and sleeping well. All of which I have had issues with most of my 60 years of life.

— *Ann Torruellas, Tempe, AZ*

Hip Pain and Work Stress Released

I have been having pain in my right hip for four months. I used Belly Button Healing to release tension (9 o'clock direction), and it relieved the pain significantly. And I use Belly Button Healing to release tension from work stress. My friend has been trying this too, and he's been going to the bathroom more frequently and felt more relaxed.

— *Chun Mu, Duluth, GA*

New Habit of Checking My Health Condition

I've normally felt that I don't have much of a problem with my health. Even so, I've been gradually doing Belly Button Healing more often. This is because, when my head feels heavy or tense for some reason, I feel my condition changing if I do Belly Button Healing even for just a moment. My head feels lighter as my body soon grows warmer and my tension is released. The places where I feel pain when I use the Belly Button Healing Wand differ according to the condition of my body. I made up my mind to make a habit of checking my condition and releasing stress on a daily basis, and I always keep the Belly Button Healing Wand close by and use it often.

— *Jiyeon Lee, South Korea*

My Body Warmed Up

I had a tugging sensation in my left side at my waist when I pressed my navel for the first time, and my hands and feet tingled, as if cold energy was leaving my body. The tension gradually released as I did Belly Button Healing, and then warm energy started circulating in my body and my hands and feet also began to warm up. I experienced my abdomen becoming really comfortable and my head really clear after five minutes of Belly Button Healing.

– Minseon Song, South Korea

Body Feels Like New

My lower back has always caused me trouble since I sprained it during gym class in junior high school. Unable to move my lower back as I'd like, I found that my intestines became stiff and that I had problems with bowel movements. My liver, which processes waste products and toxins, also had a hard time of it, and my head often felt heavy and numb.

What broke this chain of reactions in my body was Belly Button Healing. It relaxes my intestines centered on my navel, so my lower back has felt more comfortable, and I've also been able to smoothly move my left shoulder, which had been a problem. I also felt a lot of heat in my body, and, more than anything else, my head has felt clear and refreshed, and I can see more clearly.

When I haven't had a Belly Button Healing Wand near-by, I've done Belly Button Healing whenever I've had the op-portunity during the day by using my hands or a suitable tool I've found nearby. I generally spend a lot of time seated in a chair with a bloated stomach after eating. Living this way has kept my energy and blood from circulating properly, which has caused me to be in poor physical condition. Breathing and doing Belly Button Healing, though, I've felt the waste products and toxins leaving my body. As I do Belly Button Healing, blockages in my body open up and my blood and energy circulate well, making my body feel like new and giv-ing me the sudden realization that I should manage and take care of my body.

— *Giseon Kwon, former Chief of Police, Busan, South Korea*

Tension Throughout My Body Released

Before I experienced Belly Button Healing, I thought that it might be getting acupressure on your belly button. After ex-periencing it, I was left with a strong, lingering feeling like I was connected to a "tube" by my navel, and I breathed deeply as the tension throughout my body was released. I quietly sensed my body as I focused on my breathing, and, as the cold energy in my lower body went out through my left foot, my body gradually became warmer and more comfortable.

— *Sehyeon Kim, South Korea*

Anxiety Subsided

I was feeling so much anxiety as I began Belly Button Healing. I had been caught up in the residue of emotion from an uncomfortable interaction I'd had just before. But after doing Belly Button Breathing and bringing energy down, even for a short duration, I could feel that anxiety subside, and I chose not to dwell there any longer. I was even able to experience a genuine gratitude for the previous encounter and how it actually helped me to grow. I am grateful for this method and will continue to practice with it.

— Elise Kerrigan, Arlington, MA

Less Pain and Anxiety, More Calm and Energy

My reactions to a few minutes of Belly Button Healing on myself may seem insignificant, but in fact are very significant to my emotional and physical health. Almost always, I am aware that Belly Button Healing relaxes my lower back so that there is almost no feeling of pain. Only occasionally am I restricted in my daily life by the lower back pain, but so much of my body is often tense. The tenseness goes up and down my spine and into my right shoulder. Relaxing the lower back has an expanding effect. Also, I occasionally experience anxiety and an active mind. Yesterday afternoon, I did Belly Button Healing when I felt suddenly anxious, and the feeling almost completely disappeared, leaving me calm and energized to continue the day. So little effort for such great results!

— *Ann Tognetti, Gaithersburg, MD*

Helped Me Cope with Vertigo

I have been having vertigo and not been able to lie down flat on my back as the room would spin, so I would lie down on my side and was doing my Belly Button Healing with the Healing Life wand on my side. I was not pushing hard though I was doing constant pressure for about 10 minutes. At one point in the healing, I felt my ear drain down the back of my throat. I could tell it was this because the fluid that came down the back of my throat had a metallic taste so it was not regular saliva. And since then, I have not experienced any vertigo! The human body is amazing! Who would ever imagine that my ear is connected in some mystical way to my belly button.

— *Stephanie Wilson, Phoenix, AZ*

AFTERWORD
Three Times a Day

We live in space and time. To really live our lives well, we should check ourselves to see whether we are making good use of that space and time or just spending our days under their domination. You can create a satisfying, fulfilling life if you are able to design and use your space and time in the way you want.

How do you begin and end your day? Most people begin their day hating to wake up in the morning, and they go to sleep after a hard day without cleansing their emotions. Those who have jobs tend to live their lives controlled by time, as, out of obligation, they check the clock for the time to go to work, the time of their next meeting, and the time to get off work.

Communication with yourself is more important than anything else for actively directing your time instead of passively being led about by it. In other words, it's living each and every waking moment. For this, I want to recommend that you communicate with yourself as you do Belly Button Healing three times a day. Report to yourself, with determination and encouragement, how you will use your time going forward.

As soon as you get up in the morning, press your belly

button and do your beginning report with the attitude, "I will live today with meaning and passion, and I will make it a moving, happy day." And also make an intermediate report to yourself in the afternoon. "What have I done so far today? How will I spend the time I have left?"

And, as you close out the day, do a closing report, thinking, "How did I live today? Did I do work that was somehow meaningful?"

These are reports you make to your soul, not to anyone else. "I am now the master of my life. I will design my life." Making this resolution, remind yourself of it and encourage yourself three times each day. Through this, you will be able to communicate with and to achieve unity with yourself.

The starting point is the belly button. One minute is enough for pressing your belly button. After pressing your navel and focusing on your body while breathing for a while, your energy and blood circulation will improve, your body will become warmer, your breathing will becomes deeper, and your mood will be better than before. If you concentrate your awareness in your body as you do Belly Button Breathing, your consciousness, once harried by time or the external environment, will come into your body. In that instant, your consciousness will come back into your center, where it should have been in the first place. You will finally manifest insight, and, so, will be able to newly design your time and life, when your consciousness is centered.

Small adjustments in how you live will change your life.

As you communicate with yourself three times a day, try thinking, "How should I upgrade myself more? How can I give more hope and joy to the people around me today than I did yesterday?" Change your emotions with a bright smile even if you're not in the mood, and cheerfully greet those around you. If you do that for just a few days, people will ask you, "Has something good happened to you?" And good things will undoubtedly start to happen.

Doing Belly Button Healing three times a day is significant on more than a physical level. You can also connect with the earth as you do Belly Button Healing. Our bodies are part of nature, and the earth is nature; they are ultimately one. As you do Belly Button Healing, try to think, "I'm also healing the earth right now. Because my body is a part of the earth and for the earth." If you do this, you'll be able to feel your consciousness expanding even more.

First, try doing this for just 21 days. If you do, your life will start to change. What's really important is that your life changes substantially through practice.

Belly Button Healing three times a day! An Earth Citizen starts her day by communicating with herself as she presses her belly button. Ask your navel how you will live a life of healing, a life of creating and sharing health, happiness, and peace. You can find all the answers through your belly button.

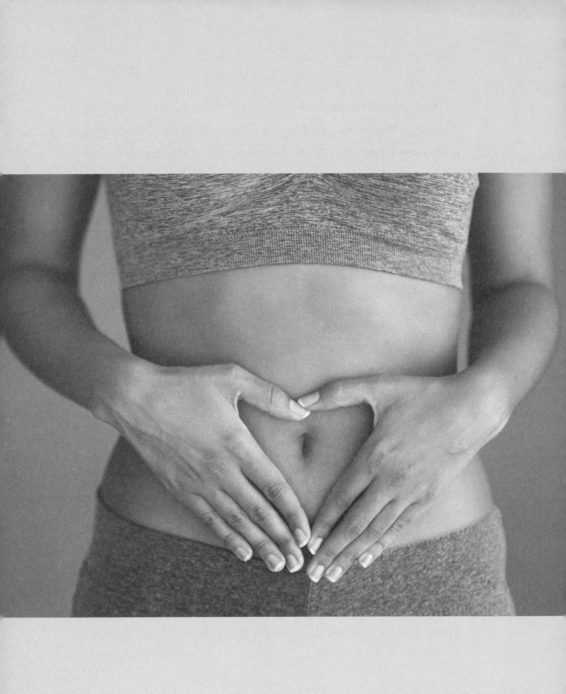

FAQ

Frequently Asked Questions About Belly Button Healing

Q: What are the main benefits of Belly Button Healing?

The most frequently reported benefits include improved digestion, stress relief, better sleep, pain relief, energy boost, and better mood. Meditators have reported being able to get into a meditative state much faster and deeper after doing Belly Button Healing.

Q: How does Belly Button Healing create such benefits?

The wide range of benefits of Belly Button Healing is possible for a very simple reason: Your belly button is the center point of your gut and your entire body. By stimulating this point, you can create positive, rippling effects in your entire body and mind from the inside out.

Just below the surface of your belly button lies an extensive "superhighway" network of nerves (vagus nerve) that works as a communication hotline between your gut and brain. Belly Button Healing's focused stimulation of the gut, practiced in conjunction with breathing, can improve the communication between your gut and brain through this super highway. Not only that, it has been shown to enhance the circulation of blood, lymph, and energy and to foster detoxification in the gut. Through this process, your body and mind are empowered to heal and return to their natural balance.

Q: How long should I do it? When? How often?

If you are new to Belly Button Healing, start slow. I recommend a slow and shallow pumping motion, about 200-300 times. That may seem like a lot but that's only about 3 minutes of practice at a rate of 100 times per minute.

How long? I recommend doing three to five minutes of varying intensity during each session.

When? Twice per day is best, once in the morning and once in the evening, to wake the body up and then to get ready for a deep and restful sleep. Many people find it very effective to include Belly Button Healing in their morning and evening exercise routines. You can also do Belly Button Healing any time during the day if you become stressed, tired, or uninspired, or if you experience any type of pain.

How often? This really depends on your needs, wants, and time availability. I believe it is best to experience Belly Button

Healing daily on a regular schedule, but everyone's capabilities will vary. An easy way to gauge your needs is to start with three minutes in the morning and three minutes in the evening. This will give you a good idea of how that amount of time makes you feel and what you need to make any adjustments. Once you feel comfortable with this schedule, you can add sessions during the middle of the day or as needed. You can also increase the time of each session up to 10-15 minutes if needed. However often you perform Belly Button Healing, always finish with slow, deep breathing for five minutes.

Q: Is it really safe to put pressure on my belly button?

Yes, as long as you follow the guidelines. At first, you might feel discomfort as you push on your belly button because of natural tension from never being touched. Go slow, listen to your body, and breathe out naturally as you push in. As you get used to it, you will feel the tension release and a wave of peace and comfort flow over your body. Many doctors are using Belly Button Healing or themselves and are also recommending it to their patients to help improve their health condition. Please consult with your doctor if you have any health concerns before starting Belly Button Healing.

Q: What is the best way to breathe during Belly Button Healing?

Exhaling in sharp, short breaths through the mouth with each press into your belly button is one of the main ways to breathe suggested for Belly Button Healing. However, this method can be difficult for some people and can become tiring over long periods of time. What's important is following your own body's natural rhythm and releasing stagnant energy and tension by breathing out through the mouth. Simply breathe naturally with your mouth slightly open instead of focusing on breathing too much.

Q: Is it okay for people with a hernia to do Belly Button Healing?

A hernia happens when the intestines bulge out of the abdominal cavity due to weak abdominal muscles. I wouldn't recommend pressing on the hernia area with the Belly Button Healing wand, because it might cause some injury. Instead, do gentle intestinal exercise or abdominal breathing.

Q: Is it safe to do Belly Button Healing if I have bladder or kidney problems?

Generally speaking, doing Belly Button Healing can increase blood flow to the internal organs and help remove toxins faster. I've heard many anecdotal stories of people who improved bladder and kidney issues by using Belly Button Healing. But, if you have had a surgical procedure done on your bladder or around that region, please consult with your doctor first.

Q: Is it okay to do Belly Button Healing during my period or if I have menstrual cramps?

The abdomen is cold when you have menstrual cramps. Increasing circulation by stimulating the abdominal area could help with menstrual cramps. However, if you are bleeding heavily, you should be gentle when doing Belly Button Healing.

Q: Is it okay to do Belly Button Healing if I wear a pacemaker?

A pacemaker is activated when your heart rate slows down. Exercises that enhance your circulation generally increase your heart rate. It's always safest to consult with your doctor first if you have any medical concerns. You should not tap over the pacemaker area with the Belly Button Healing wand, as it might activate the device.

Q: I have recently had surgery. Is it safe to use?

I recommend getting the opinion of your medical doctor or surgeon before using Belly Button Healing after a surgery. Different parts of the body heal at a various times and may need more rest. Although you feel energized and healed, stimulating the abdomen could have a negative effect on your healing, depending on where you had surgery. When you do begin performing Belly Button Healing, be very aware of how your body reacts and what it is telling you.

Q: What's the difference between using the Belly Button Healing wand vs. my fingers or other instruments?

One of the key features of the Belly Button Healing wand's design is the ergonomic shape. The T-shape allows you to perform Belly Button Healing easily without strain to your shoulders, neck, or arms. You can also alter the pressure you place on your navel with the different sized ends to be gentle or firm, without much difference in physical effort, because of the unique shape. It also can be used more effectively on other parts of your body, giving you stronger and more targeted stimulation with greater reach. You can absolutely use your fingers or some other similar object to perform Belly Button Healing, but the results and efficiency will vary.

Acknowledgments

I would like to extend my sincere gratitude to all who have contributed to the creation of this book. Hyerin Moon, Jiyoung Oh, and Michela Mangiaracina at Best Life Media, Steve Kim, and the staff of Hanmunhwa Multimedia tirelessly helped me, from the original research and writing, to editing, to the final production. I am grateful for their dedicated editorial support.

I would like to thank Daniel Graham for helping transform my Korean into English, and Nicole Dean for polishing it further. I also extend great thanks to Jooyoung Ryu for the illustrations and to Kiryl Lysenka for his creative design of the cover.

Special thanks to Janet Mills, the co-author of *The Four Agreements*, for reading the manuscript and adding her valuable insights. I would also like to thank Dr. James Westphal, Dr. Reed Tuckson, Dr. Edward Jang, and Dr. Deborah Coady, who passionately endorsed *Belly Button Healing*.

Resources

If you want more instruction in Belly Button Healing, or if you want ways to apply it, you can find them both offline and online from the following resources.

BellyButtonHealing.com

A one-stop space for all things related to Belly Button Healing, visit this site to find more how-tos, advice, and workshops, or to purchase online courses or Belly Button Healing tools. This website will be updated on an ongoing basis as more resources are made.

Body & Brain Yoga and Tai Chi

Find experienced instructors in Belly Button Healing and other healthy belly exercises at approximately 100 Body & Brain centers around the United States. Have them check the energetic condition of your gut, and help you tailor Belly Button Healing to your individual lifestyle. The dedicated mentors at the Body & Brain centers will personally guide you in using Belly Button Healing as the starting point to making the changes you want in your life. Body & Brain centers have been teaching Ilchi Lee's self-healing methods in the U.S. for over 20 years and are found in many major cities. Search for one near you at **www.bodynbrain.com**.

ChangeYourEnergy.com

A multimedia educational site founded by Ilchi Lee, ChangeYourEnergy.com has a wide variety of online courses, articles, and videos, as well as offline tools, for personal development. Their unique and ever-growing offerings help you explore and enhance your body's energy system and use it to bloom every part of your life. Look for practical advice on how to keep your gut, and your life, healthy and happy.

Earth Citizens Organization

Belly Button Healing users often find themselves wanting to act to help other people and the earth be healthier. The Earth Citizens Organization (ECO) is the hub of the Earth Citizen Movement in the United States. This nonprofit founded by Ilchi Lee trains leaders in mindful and sustainable living and aids them in sharing that in their communities. People who have declared themselves Earth Citizens are gathering to raise public awareness for sustainability, teach mind-body exercises, and engage community actions for positive changes. For tips on how to live mindfully and sustainably and find out more about the Earth Citizen Movement in your community, visit **www.earthcitizens.org**.